Living Light

The 21-Day Alchemical Regeneration Plan

Chavah Aima

ENLIGHTENED LIFE PUBLISHING
AUSTIN, TEXAS, U.S.A.

Copyright © 2007 by Chavah Aima

All rights reserved. No part of this book may be reproduced or transmitted in any form or by any means, electronic or mechanical, including photocopying, recording, or by any information storage and retrieval system, without permission in writing from the Publisher. Reviewers may quote brief passages.

Enlightened Life Publishing
P.O. Box 82242
Austin, TX 78708
U.S.A.
www.enlightenedlife.org

ISBN 978-0-9705518-2-5

Book Design, Layout, and Cover Art by Artline Graphics, Sedona Arizona

Alchemical Drawings and Yoga Illustrations by Maryam Ahmed, scorpio1576@yahoo.com

Alchemical Meditation Illustrations by New Way Solutions, www.newwaysolutions.com

Thanks to:

Hira Ratan Manek for permission to summarize his work with Solar Gazing, www.solarhealing.com

Andre Le Verre for permission to use his painting, *Let there be Light*, which appears on page 55 www.contemplative-art.com

Robert Frost for permission to use his photographs of his garden, www.joyousworld.com

Publishers Note

Nothing in this book is intended to constitute medical advice or to diagnose or treat any disease or illness. Before beginning any diet or exercise program you should consult with your health care professional, and follow his/her advice. As each individual is unique, the reader is advised to use their discretion in applying the principles and program components described in this book. The natural food diet suggested herein is meant to provide nutritional support only, and is not a substitute for drugs, surgery, or medical treatment. Your health and well-being are your responsibility, and if you have any medical problems or suspect that you may have a medical problem, we urge you to seek professional advice immediately. Neither the publisher nor the author shall be liable or responsible for any problems allegedly arising from any information or suggestion in this book.

Table of Contents

Introduction	1
Chapter 1: Seven Keys to Radiant Health and Spiritual Abundance	7
Chapter 2: Getting Ready to Regenerate	35
Chapter 3: Program Schedule and Menu Plans	57
Chapter 4: Living Light Recipes	75
Chapter 5: Alchemical Yoga: Living Light Meditations	117
Chapter 6: Alchemical Yoga: Breath and Movement	143
Chapter 7: Beyond Living Light	163
Appendix	181
Endnotes	186
Bibliography	192
Index	195
About the Author	200

Acknowledgements

I am grateful for the inspirational instruction of many teachers and masters in the Western and Eastern traditions of enlightenment, especially Florence Farr, Moina and Samuel Mathers, Paul Foster Case, Dr. Israel Regardie, Swami Muktananda, Hira Ratan Manek, Edmond Bordeaux Szekely, Viktoras Kulvinskas, Yogi Bhajan, Ramana Maharshi, Mouni Saddhu, and Reverend Russell Nees. I am also indebted to the wise and invisible guides of the inner planes who continue to clarify my understandings and direct my work.

I appreciate the assistance of my daughter Elizabeth Stewart for her initial consultation and editing of the book. Special thanks to Mike Jung for his expert advice and design concepts. I am especially grateful to my beloved partner Evan Mills for his valuable assistance with every aspect of the book, and for his patience, love, and ongoing support of my life-work.

Dedication

This book is dedicated to the divine being
that lies within your human form.
May it awaken fully and live freely.

Introduction

My experience with living foods and juices began twenty years ago when I was a member of a meditation group hosted by Reverend Russell Nees and his wife Mary Helon. Russell was a professor of parapsychology at the University of Texas. In addition to other things, they taught me the Essene approach to healing and regeneration, which is inspired by a deep realization of the sacred powers inherent in natural, living foods. They went on to establish the Optimum Health Institute in Austin, Texas, where I had the opportunity to meet and learn from Viktoras Kulvinskas, who is in many ways the founding father of the modern raw food movement.

At the time my path crossed with these Essene mentors, I was working as a professional psychotherapist specializing in the treatment of psychological trauma, addiction, and compulsive behavior. I was also deeply involved in the study and practice of the ageless wisdom traditions of Kabbalah, Rosicrucianism, and Alchemy. As the occult psychology of these ancient disciplines merged with my clinical practice, I was able to offer my clients an expanded awareness of the true nature and purpose of life's challenges. My counseling sessions were marked by the frequent intervention of angelic beings and the appearance of radiant light, which often brought about spontaneous healing. These powerful experiences led me away from the limited understandings and methods of clinical psychology into the superior, holistic approaches of esoteric, spiritual psychology.

During a long period of isolated spiritual practice and intensive meditation, I experienced the *illumination* of Alchemy, which induced expanded states of consciousness and brought forth radical personal transformations and greater alignment with the higher self. My understanding of the esoteric arts and sciences crystallized, and became integrated as deep cellular wisdom. During this time I also received the inner initiations of the true Rosicrucian order that operates upon the invisible planes. I traveled to India where I experienced the awakening of the Kundalini, the *Vital Essence* within. On journeys to Europe, I spent time with sages of the Western esoteric traditions, and was led into profound initiatory experiences.

Many of the teachings of Alchemy mirror the principles found in the Eastern philosophies of Kundalini and Tantra yoga. These paths offer techniques that bring one into greater awareness of the cosmic energy that underlies creation. Alchemists refer to this energy as spiritual *light*, the source vibration of all that exists. This light resides in abundance in the living plants of the earth and sea, and also lies deep within a secret reservoir in the human body. When it is accessed consciously it may be used to bring about healing, emotional transmutation, and the illumination of the mind. Alchemists work to increase its availability through diet, breath-work, meditation, and other methods. As their command of the light strengthens, they are able to effect deeper transformations and more rapid manifestations.

The alchemist also makes use of the powers of the imagination and will, strengthening them greatly on the quest for spiritual life. Alchemical meditation focuses primarily on light energy, which is visualized within and around the physical body. Specific structures and forms are created with the imagination, and anchored by the will into the *etheric body*, the energy field in which the physical, mental, and emotional bodies reside. Mastery of the etheric plane allows the practitioner to create and manifest selected conditions in the body and the world.

The first stages of alchemical *light work* involve the removal of impurities and imbalances that affect all things

Introduction

in the material world, and in particular the physical body. The body is the *vessel* in which the *Great Art* of regeneration occurs. The cells become purified through preliminary disciplines during which more light is consciously taken in. Alchemy refers us to the foods and substances that offer the most light: the living plants of the earth and their juices. Beyond the application of light toward the cleansing and healing of the body and persona lie the greater mystical promises of Alchemy: abundant health, spiritual powers, longevity, and even immortality.

As I began to blend the philosophy and practices of the alchemists and yogi's, I was aware that the divine life promised by these ancient traditions can only come about when combined with the healing and regenerative powers of raw foods, juices, and fasting. The ancient alchemical texts and symbols are filled with subtle references to diet and internal cleansing as key components of the *Great Art*. In light of this knowledge, I developed a 21-day fast using a raw food diet and organic juices, which I first introduced to my students who were also involved in an ongoing program of daily alchemical meditation, Kabbalah study, ceremonials, and regular yoga practice. For several years this program has been used with extraordinary success by my students around the world.

In addition to teaching esoteric arts and sciences, I also continued to consult with people facing personal challenges ranging from obesity to depression. I often directed them to try an 80 to 100% raw food diet combined with fasting on juices, alchemical meditation, and yoga. The results were dramatic and included increased energy, more effective detoxification, visible reversal of aging, and lasting shifts in consciousness. However, without the key practices of Alchemy, the changes induced by diet alone were often undone by subtle influences from the subconscious mind. Alchemical meditation realigns the physical body with the etheric body, and helps transmute unconscious mental and emotional patterns while strengthening and clarifying one's connection to the soul.

Ultimately my work in merging these powerful disciplines became known as Alchemical Yoga®, a holistic path encompassing self-improvement, a healthy lifestyle, and the possibility of extraordinary spiritual attainment. It is a modern spiritual technology for advancing human potentials that can be used in conjunction with any religion or philosophy, or with none. To apply its methods for the healing and regeneration of the physical body requires no special knowledge of Kabbalah, Alchemy, or Yoga. *Alchemical Yoga* is a divine science that stimulates and sustains positive, inspired growth in every aspect of one's life.

Living Light: The 21-day Alchemical Regeneration Plan is a modified version of the program that I first designed for my students. The Living Light plan can be used two to three times a year as an overall cleansing and rejuvenation program, or it can serve as a way to successfully transition into an 80 to 100% raw food diet. Special alchemical meditations and yoga exercises have been designed for Living Light and form an integral part of the plan. These practices accelerate healing by increasing and intensifying light energy within the body, mind, and soul. They are easy to learn and can be used safely by everyone.

As you begin the Living Light program, take time to read and contemplate the information in each chapter. Chapter One describes seven keys that lead to radiant health and spiritual life. This overview introduces some of the essential secrets of Alchemy, giving insight into simple lifestyle practices that can lead to extraordinary transformation. The remaining chapters provide the details of the Living Light plan, including program schedules, sample menus, buying and producing living foods, delicious recipes, and the empowering meditations and practices of *Alchemical Yoga*.

For those who have already embraced a raw food diet, the Living Light plan offers special alchemical techniques that can magnify and focus the light energy being received through one's food, and many delightful new recipes. If your raw food journey begins with Living Light, please don't let it end there. Use the program frequently to cleanse and renew your body, mind, and soul. Once you have experienced the phenomenal rewards that come from Living Light, you may decide to join the multitude of people all over the world who are living and thriving on raw foods. There are many resources for support to continue with the raw food lifestyle, some of which are highlighted in the Appendix.

Introduction

Further education and experience with the unique fusion of Eastern and Western spiritual technologies that I offer are available through Alchemical Yoga. My work also continues to evolve through Enlightened Life Sanctuary, an international non-profit organization that encourages the wise use of our collective spiritual and material resources to consciously create sustainable and enlightened life on earth.

I wish you great success with Living Light, and all the best that life has to offer always!

Chavah Aima
Sedona Arizona
August 2007

Chapter One

Seven Keys
To Radiant Health
and Spiritual Abundance

THE GUIDING PRINCIPLES
OF THE LIVING LIGHT PROGRAM

There are a wide variety of ancient spiritual philosophies that give advice for recovering health and regenerating the physical body. The inspirational principles that form the foundation of the Living Light program are drawn from the ageless wisdom of the Essenes, Alchemy, Yoga, the Egyptian Rosicrucian traditions, Kabbalah, and Esoteric Psychology. The sacred keys derived from these sources promise radiant physical health and vitality. Used wisely, they can open interior gateways and lead one into the eternal source of pure understanding.

The treasured concepts and practices of these traditions have been upheld by modern science as being essential for health and highly useful for healing a variety of disorders. Living Light focuses on seven wisdom principles and integrates them in a 21-day program that will detoxify and regenerate body, mind, and soul. These components are: *Vital Essence*, a natural living food diet, juice fasting, sunshine, meditation, breath and movement, and joy. The teachings and practices behind each key principle are introduced below, and expanded upon throughout the program chapters that follow.

The First Key: Vital Essence

In Alchemy, *Vital Essence* is the endless energy that creates and sustains the universe. It is always available everywhere – in sunshine, air, water, food, trees, earth, plants, and within all sentient beings. It can be accessed in greater quantity when one is mindful of its presence. This is the energy that gives life to everything that lives. Vital Essence is a conscious, invisible force that initiates and permeates all of creation.

Vital Essence is known by many names in the various spiritual cultures of the world. The Taoists call it Chi, and have charts depicting its flow through the body. Indian Yogi's refer to it as Prana, which they use for healing and miracles. The Polynesian shamans call it Mana, and they extract it from rocks, plants, air, and water for use in healing and magic. In Japan it is known as Ki, the energy used in Reiki healing. Dr. Wilhelm Reich discovered this force in the human body, and called it Orgone energy. He created a type of psychotherapy that increases this energy, causing the breakdown and release of old emotional patterns held within the body. In Kabbalah, Vital Essence is known as Chiyah, the Living Light that emanates from the realm of the cosmic father to begin and sustain creation.

An adequate influx of Vital Essence into the body is required for good health. This essence is the force that spins the chakras of the subtle body, providing the electrical current that drives human life. It powers every aspect of the body – cells, nerves, blood, tissues, and bones. The amount of Vital Essence in the body determines the degree of health, youthfulness, and vibrancy one experiences. Sickness and disease are symptoms of an insufficient flow of this essential energy. Vital Essence is the key element that brings health, happiness, and success into one's life.

The amount of available Vital Essence is limitless. In the physical world of creation it is hard to imagine the concept of *limitlessness*. Yet, this is the true nature of this cosmic force. Though it is endless, the available quantity of Vital Essence is typically limited by restrictions in the physical body, conditioned mental patterns, and unresolved emotional issues. The esoteric systems of Kabbalah and Alchemy offer a holistic spiritual psychology that can help free one from such obstacles.

Vital Essence within the body-mind organism can be built up through many methods. One may experience a surge of Vital Essence by consciously connecting with the sacred powers of fire, water, earth, and air found within all of nature. Evergreens are especially high in this living energy and one's strength and stamina may be renewed by spending time in a forest.[1] Breathing practices, physical exercise, and yoga as described in the Sixth Key below, also stimulate and increase Vital Essence within the physical body.

The sun is the most prolific provider of Vital Essence on the earth. This is why people feel happier and brighter on sunny days than they do on rainy days. The force is more directly available during the day than it is at night when it flows more subtly. Solar gazing and sun bathing allow one to absorb more Vital Essence directly from the sun. Greater solar radiance may also be attained by conscious connection with the sun through meditation, prayer, and ceremony. Many of these methods are highlighted in the Fourth Key below.

Vital Essence is the driving force behind all thoughts, emotions, and physical expressions. One of its most vigorous manifestations is sexual energy. In this aspect, it gives a couple the awesome power to bring forth human life. There is a reservoir of cosmic Vital Essence that lies coiled at the base of the spine, and remains dormant in most people. This secret reserve is known as *Kundalini* in the Eastern spiritual traditions, while the alchemists of the West call it *Serpent Power*.

Awakening, activating, and raising the Serpent can bring about cosmic consciousness, and firmly establish one's own spiritual authority as the primary director of life. Sometimes the Serpent awakens spontaneously, stimulating psychic and spiritual powers, which may cause distress or be misunderstood. Generally, one must work consciously to rouse the force, or receive an activating transmission through a teacher, group, or spiritual master.

When the Serpent remains in the lower chakras, the energy manifests primarily as sexuality, aggression, and ambition. The alchemist consciously works to cleanse and balance the body and mind before awakening the force. The energy is then transmuted as it flows upward into the heart chakra where the vibration begins to manifest as purified love. This accomplishment instills deep serenity and a more detached, compassionate outlook on life.

In the higher stages of alchemical transformation the Serpent may rise again, strengthening intuitive powers such as clairvoyance and telepathy. Cosmic consciousness may be realized when the energy lifts beyond the top of the head. The alchemist redirects this upward flow back into the bottom chakra to create a circle of eternal energy within the body. This attainment is represented in alchemical symbolism by the *Ouroboros*, a Serpent eating its own tail.

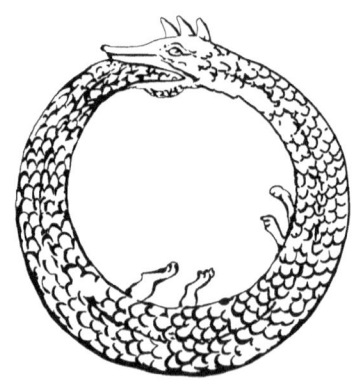

"Kundalini is one of the greatest energies.
The whole body of the seeker starts glowing
because of the rising of the Kundalini."
Gyaneshwari, Chapter VI

Methods for Increasing Vital Essence

- Consume fresh organic juices, raw fruits and vegetables, seeds, nuts, and all living foods.
- Absorb solar radiance through solar gazing, sun bathing, and meditation on the sun.
- Spend time in nature. Hike, camp, and consciously communicate with plants, trees, rocks, streams, rivers, air, wind, and sea. Humbly ask for more energy from nature, and receive it with love and gratitude.
- Learn and practice *Alchemical Yoga®*[2], Hatha Yoga, or Kundalini Yoga.
- Meditate on the sexual energy in your body, consciously moving it upward until you can feel it as intensely in the higher chakras as you can in the lower ones. Practice this technique alone and with your intimate partner.
- Study and explore the healing technologies of Alchemy, Qi Gong, Tao, Reiki, Kahuna, Bioenergetics, Kabbalah, Yoga, and other disciplines that consciously access and direct Vital Essence.

The Second Key: A Natural Living Food Diet

"I give you every plant and fruit bearing tree
for food and for medicine."
Genesis

The ancient alchemists were wise men and women who knew the powerful mysteries of spiritual transformation. They often hid their secrets with confusing words and symbolic images. Modern alchemists understand that the physical body is the *vessel* in which the sacred metamorphosis from natural human to divine being occurs. In Alchemy, enlightenment is a physiological process that may culminate in great spiritual attainment. The key to this mechanism lies within the digestive track and depends upon the quality of the vibratory energy that enters into the body via food and drink.

    Certain foods, particularly processed food, meat, and dairy products, cannot be easily digested and eliminated by the human body, and may remain in the digestive track for years, fermenting and rotting. These undigested remnants become an underlying source of many diseases, ill health, and a shortened life. The decomposing remains of animal flesh, which become trapped in the bowel, can attract invisible dark entities to cohabitate in the body. These ethereal beings can be thought of as *alchemical demons* that limit one's consciousness, and offer openings into the human form for pain, disease, and death.

In the body, these demons transmute into carcinogens and free radicals, which cause cancer and disrupt the systems that are vital to good health. Their presence is insidious, and they encourage troublesome habits and the consumption of more bad foods. These subtle forces are also often at the core of addictions, compulsions, and eating disorders.

Alchemical texts refer to this state of corrupted health as the *black dragon of putrefaction*.[3] This condition of bodily contamination was diagnosed when the noxious decayed matter within the body was expelled from the bowels as dark, foul excrement. However, in Alchemy, equilibrium is the secret to accomplishing the *Great Art* of transformation, and favorable conditions may be restored by applying correct methods.

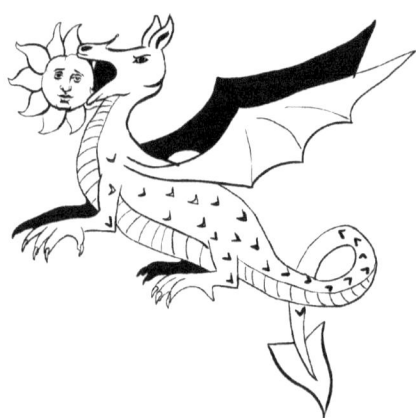

This Green-Dragon is the natural Gold of the Philosophers...
without the true knowledge and right Manipulation
of it nothing can be done in our Art.

Alchemists also describe a *green dragon* that is the *natural gold* of the alchemists.[4] The green dragon symbolizes the living plants of the earth that contain the energy of the sun. These are the foods that can purify, heal, and cleanse the body of leftover wastes, which in turn causes the demons to flee. Raw and living foods and juices are filled with all of the Vital Essence of nature. These substances attract *alchemical angels* into the body, which manifest as antioxidants, white blood cells, vital nutrients, and oxygen. These angels lift one's spirits and help maintain radiant health.

In the Rosicrucian view, the human being falls away from his/her true divine state due to the many negative influences that exist within the material world. These effects come in the form of emotions, thoughts, food, and toxic environments. Rising from this fall involves a complete detoxification from negative emotions, erroneous beliefs, and deadly foods. As deep cleansing takes place, the higher self may reintegrate with the physical body. This process is known as *regeneration*, and it may be repeated many times to bring one into ever-improving states of health and well being.

The alchemists looked at every level of being, and also addressed the spiritual benefits that may come from consciously applying alchemical dietary and meditative practices toward the creation of an immortal body. Those who desire greater health as well as those who seek divine illumination should carefully consider the powerful impact natural living food has in the accomplishment of these goals. The Vital Essence of the sun transmutes into a special nutritional form within each plant, and one seeking to heal and enlighten the body-mind organism makes wise use of this truth of nature.

When a pure diet of raw foods is eaten, a process of deep transformation takes place in the body, mind, and soul. As the body becomes filled with angels, one may experience increased psychic and spiritual sensitivity. One who perseveres in the process of regeneration may naturally become a healing presence for others as the body becomes more subtle and offers less resistance to divine vibrations.

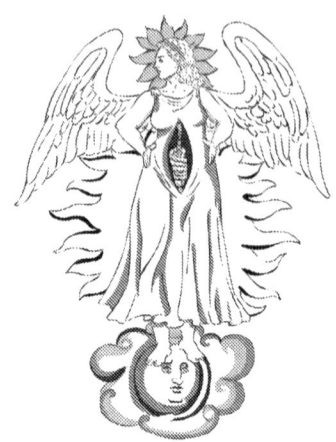

The Alchemists' Secret:
Absorbing solar radiance through conscious digestion

Eating food in its natural state is superior in every way to eating food that has been modified, processed, chemically treated, and/or cooked. Organic living foods should ideally form 60-90% of a healthy person's diet. In certain diseases and illnesses, all cooked food should be avoided.

The vegetarian and vegan diets have been proven many times to improve health and lengthen life. The diseases now linked to eating meat are too numerous to list. For example, one U.S. study found that eliminating meat and dairy products from the diet reduced heart attack risk by 90%.[5]

Animals are sentient creatures and science shows that even fish feel pain when they are caught.[6] The cells of the body are formed from the food one eats. Animal flesh holds the vibrations of the great fear and stress that the animal suffered during the horrific circumstances of its death. It is best to eat a vegan diet which brings the vibrations of compassion, non-violence, and unity into the physical form.

Plants are also living entities. Spiritually, plants can be viewed as special intelligences whose purpose is to manifest as unique, edible forms of vital solar force. They are divine agents who freely distribute superior nutrition and alchemical nectar to humans. In the Essene traditions, plants are said to be attended by loving angels. Communion prayers to these angels are recited at mealtimes and throughout the day to acknowledge and connect with the spiritual consciousness that resides in the sun, air, earth, and plants.

The advantages of the raw food diet are many. In 1940, Dr. E.B. Szekely, who introduced *The Essene Gospels*, founded a healing center in Mexico based on the dietary principles described in the Gospels. Over the next thirty years at Rancho La Puerta Retreat more than 120,000 people experienced a 90% recovery rate from all types of health problems, including cancer, by following an 80-100% live-vegetarian diet.[7] Rancho La Puerta inspired the creation of many other Essene-based residential detoxification and healing programs throughout the world that have seen similar results.

The Living Light plan was inspired by the wisdom teachings of Alchemy and the remarkable healing experiences of multitudes of people who have benefited from raw food healing programs. It has been designed to help you gain all of the rewards offered by a raw food diet, and it also includes key secrets of the alchemists that restore balance and accelerate regeneration. A summary of ways to get the most from the Living Light program is provided at the end of this chapter.

The Third Key: Fasting

Fasting has been used for centuries to restore and maintain health. The process of fasting not only detoxifies the body it also relieves mental and emotional stress. Various fasting methods have been successful in healing critical illnesses, diseases, depression, and addictions. Regular fasting also offers a highly effective weight loss strategy. Fasting is associated with traditional religious observances and can bring about states of greater spiritual clarity.

Fasting is best defined as abstaining from any food for a period of time. For example, if one chooses to eliminate meat from the diet for a time and later return to eating it, this is termed fasting from meat. If one does not return to eating meat, this constitutes a dietary change to vegetarianism. Living Light is a special 21-day fast that excludes meat, dairy, cooked, and processed foods, and incorporates a weekly 24-hour fast from all solid foods. Living Light can be used as a regular cleansing fast two to four times a year. The diet may also be lengthened or continued, and can serve as a gateway into raw veganism.

Fasting was among the earliest methods of healing discovered by humanity. In ancient times, members of the Essene community were widely known for their wisdom and healing abilities. They healed through natural hygiene methods, the core of which was fasting from all solid foods. As with many spiritual peoples, they also fasted as a form of communion with the divine. In the *Essene Gospel of Peace*, Jesus explained to the sick people who had gathered to fast that the allegory of the prodigal son[8] contained a secret promise of healing:

"The seven years of eating and drinking and riotous living are the sins of the past. The wicked creditor is Satan. The debts are diseases. The heavy labor is pains. The prodigal son, he is yourselves. The payment of debts is the casting from you of…diseases, and the healing of your body.

"…I tell you truly, your heavenly Father loves you without end, for he also allows you to pay in seven days the debts of seven years. Those that owe the sins and diseases of seven years, but pay honestly (by fasting) and persevere to the seventh day, to them shall our Heavenly Father forgive the debts of all these seven years."[9]

According to this teaching of Jesus, fasting for seven days can alleviate seven year's worth of the effects of unnatural living such as eating high quantities of meats and processed foods, overindulgence in food, alcohol, prescription or non-prescription drugs, environmental toxins, and pollution. The healing fast that Jesus prescribed in the *Essene Gospel of Peace* consisted of water and wheat grass juice, a serious fast that can cause severe cleansing reactions for modern people due to their higher levels of toxicity. Fasting for seven days or longer on fresh organic fruit and vegetable juices is a safe and highly beneficial alternative to water fasting, and can also be used to help one prepare for a water-only fast.

Living for a time only on juices allows one to directly partake of the high levels of Vital Essence that reside within the fruits of the earth. Juice fasting provides pure, high-powered nutrition while allowing the bodily systems to rest, cleanse, and rejuvenate. While each fruit and vegetable contains unique nutritional properties, green juices are particularly important in the alchemical process of regeneration.

The juice extracted from green vegetables, sprouts, and cereal grasses contains the greatest abundance of chlorophyll available from the plants of the earth. Chlorophyll is sunlight that has been transmuted through a natural alchemical process into an edible form. In alchemical terms, it has become the *blood* of the plant, the vital fluid that is extracted through juicing. As this liquid is consumed, the body becomes charged with the life-giving powers of the sun. The solar force is of special significance in the alchemical art of self-transformation, which is further explained in the Fourth Key below.

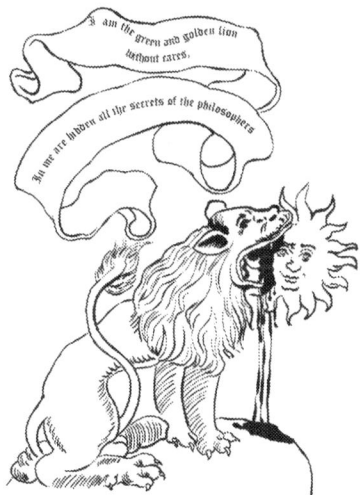

The Green Lion of Alchemy represents green plants absorbing solar power, and converting it into blood, the juice of the plant. When the human consumes green juices, the blood within the body becomes super-charged with the life-giving powers of the sun.

In the form of fresh juices, the living essence of the sun first purifies and then regenerates the cells of the body. Juice fasting increases the alkalinity of the body, an important factor in good health. The typical Western diet is overly acidic, creating an environment in the body that is the breeding ground for all disease. Restoring the body to a proper acid-alkaline balance is accomplished by increasing one's intake of alkaline foods and juices. The dark green grasses and vegetables are among the most alkaline foods, reflecting again the insightful wisdom of the ancient alchemists.

To get the most from fasting use a transitional fasting plan to ease the body into the process and lessen detoxification symptoms. Start with a one-day per week juice fast for four to six weeks. Then lengthen one of the weekly juice fasts to three days. Again in four to six weeks, fast for five days. When you are ready, undertake a seven to ten day juice fast.

Each individual will have a unique experience when fasting. When first beginning a fasting program it is wise to consult with a health care professional to address any imbalances or pre-existing conditions that may require adjustments to typical fasting protocols. If special medical conditions are present one should consult his or her health care provider before and during a fast.

To prepare juice, use a juicer that produces living juice. Living juice contains all of the vital enzymes, vitamins, and minerals of the plant. The best juicers for extracting living juice are known as *triturating* or *masticating* juicers. Such juicers produce virtually no heat, and use a slow speed to extract the juice. This type of juicer gently crushes the plant, retaining all of the vital nutritional components that may be lost in high-speed centrifugal juicers which create excessive friction and heat. Resources for juicers that produce high quality juice are listed in the Appendix.

A 30 to 90 day juice fast containing large amounts of green vegetable juice can be very beneficial in restoring health, and offers a superior weight loss program for those who are ready. However, if your diet has been very poor, or you consume large amounts of meat, dairy, alcohol, drugs, and/or junk foods, or if any special health issues exist, you should consult with a natural health care professional for specific guidance in long term juice fasting.

Water fasting is also a powerful healing method; however, most people need to prepare carefully for a water fast by undertaking an 80-100% raw vegan diet, and a regular juice fasting program for a period of time. As one becomes more detoxified through raw food and juice cleansing, short water fasts of one to three days may also be undertaken from time to time. After toxins in the body have been reduced by an improved dietary program, one may fast on water for up to ten days. If you are interested in fasting on water alone for more than ten days, please do so only in consultation with a natural health care professional experienced in supervising water fasts.

Fasting Tips

- Meditate daily.
- Always listen to your body.
- Enjoy yoga and nature walks.
- Fast from stress as well as food.
- Read spiritually inspiring books.
- Turn off the television and avoid the news.
- Drink 1.5 to 3 liters of pure water every day.
- Soak in a hot spa or bath to aid detoxification.
- Avoid strenuous and aerobic exercise for the first 2-3 days.
- Massage and chiropractic adjustments support detoxification.
- For fasts of 3 days or more, colon hydrotherapy is recommended.
- Take herbal laxative teas or supplements, enemas, or colonics to ease detox symptoms.

Common detoxification symptoms during fasting may include headaches, sore muscles and joints, fatigue, and a lower body temperature. Rest as much as possible and wear warm socks and clothing. Take comfort in knowing that these are signs of toxins leaving your body, and that the symptoms will pass in 24 to 72 hours. If symptoms are severe or get worse, seek guidance from a natural health care professional with experience in fasting and detoxification.

The Fourth Key: Sunshine

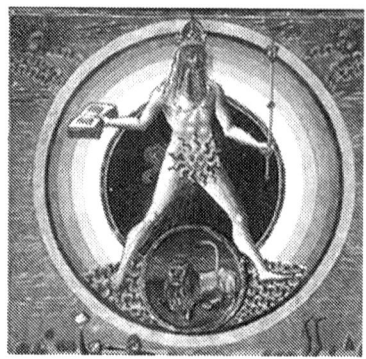

*"I am he who comes forth, opening the gates.
My will is everlasting light. I shine forth as
the Lord of Life, and the glorious law of Light."*
Egyptian Book of the Dead[10]

The sun is the source that sustains all life on earth. It provides heat and light, and also radiates cosmic force that infuses plants, animals, and humans with the energetic nutrition to grow and thrive. The Egyptians, like other ancient peoples, honored the sun for its god-like powers, which they made use of for medicine and invoked through ceremonial rites. In such rites, invocation denoted a process whereby the divine vibrations of the sun were invited to come and dwell within the body of the priest or priestess. This sacred experience of oneness with the *Lord of Life* lifted the human spirit and imbued it with supernal wisdom.

The core symbols and invocations of these ceremonials can also be effective when used in meditation. One may contact the life-giving powers of the sun through special visualizations, and receive its healing vibrations by chanting or concentrating upon key words and emblems from the ancient invocations. A weekly meditation that directly draws upon the sun's glory in such a way is included in the Living Light program.

The sun was one of the first sources that humans turned to for healing illness and disease. Modern science has now proven the ability of the sun to prevent and heal depression, vision problems, learning disabilities, and many diseases including cancer. As this book is being written, a major study has just been completed resulting in new advice from the Canadian Cancer Society that the sunshine vitamin is critical in the prevention of cancer. U.S. researchers have also found a direct link between Vitamin D deficiencies and a greatly increased incidence of cancer.

Participants in such studies take Vitamin D in supplement form, which carries the risk of toxicity if too much is consumed. The best way for humans to receive Vitamin D is by exposing the skin to sunlight. In order for the body to produce adequate levels of Vitamin D, it must be exposed to bright sunlight for a sufficient length of time each day. If one resides in a location that has only weak sunlight for long periods of time, Vitamin D supplementation may be needed.

Do not use sunscreen for your daily sunbath. Among the reasons cancer and other diseases are on the rise is the overuse of sunscreen and the avoidance of bright sun. Be aware however, that skin color and geographical location are critical factors in determining how much time is needed in the sun for the body to produce enough Vitamin D without injuring the skin. For example, dark skinned people living in far northern hemisphere locations may need much more sun exposure than light skinned people in the same area.[11]

Solar gazing offers another method for gaining additional nutrition and strength from the sun. This technique has established a history of testimony to the healing of many disorders since it was introduced to the West by Hira Ratan Manek (HRM) in 1999. HRM is a solar yogi from India whose solar gazing has enabled him to receive all of his nourishment directly from the sun. He has been observed in three medical studies abstaining from eating food for up to 411 days.

Solar gazing is done by looking at the sun as it rises or sets. One gazes for a very short time at first, incrementally increasing the length of each session over a period of nine months. Healing begins and continues as solar gazing is lengthened. Additionally, when the sun enters the visual cortex, new neural pathways are created in the brain. As more solar light is taken in, the capacity of the brain increases.

Solar gazing must be done within the first hour after sunrise or the last hour before sunset. At these times, ultraviolet rays are at their lowest levels of the day. Below is an outline of HRM's technique for solar healing.[12]

Solar Gazing Method

1. The only time solar gazing may be done safely is during the first hour after sunrise or the last hour before sunset. At these times the ultraviolet (UV) rays are very low and will not harm the eyes. Solar gazing should take place once a day every day for nine months. Choose to gaze at the sun once each day either during sunrise or sunset.

2. You must be able to see the sun on the horizon. Watching the sun set or rise behind a mountain is not advised as the UV levels are too high at these times.

3. Always stand on the earth (grass, sand, or dirt) in your bare feet while solar gazing. In cold winter climates you may remain indoors and gaze through a window.

4. On the first day, gaze at the sun for 10 seconds. On the second day look for 20 seconds. Continue to increase your viewing time by 10 seconds each day. During the first three months, you may experience cleansing symptoms as the body begins to heal and regenerate. At the end of three months, solar gazing sessions will reach 15 minutes.

5. Continue to add 10 seconds daily. During the next 90 days, the body will begin to transform the sun's rays directly into electromagnetic energy, just as the green plants synthesize sunlight. Healing will be completed, and your body will begin to store greater amounts of solar power. At the end of six months, you will be gazing at the sun for 30 minutes at a time.

6. Continue to add 10 seconds daily. Between six and nine months, you will reach 44 minutes of solar gazing daily. During this period, hunger will fade away, and your body will be able to remain healthy and highly energized without taking in food.

7. You must stop solar gazing when you reach 44 minutes. From this point on, your body can remain energized and healthy by walking barefoot on the earth for 45 minutes a day, six days a week.

Whether or not you choose to try solar gazing, be sure to expose your body to the sun daily to boost and maintain healthy levels of Vitamin D. Learn and apply the secrets of the green plants through direct alchemical synthesis, diet, and juicing. Turn the sun's power into greater Vital Essence through conscious absorption of its sacred life-giving vibrations in meditation. Light has been proclaimed to be the medicine of the future as modern physicians rediscover the ancient secrets of solar healing.

The Fifth Key: Meditation

"Know that your seeking and yearning will avail you not, unless you know the mystery: if that which you seek, you find not within yourself, you will never find it without."
The Charge of the Goddess[13]

Almost everyone has had at least a momentary experience of the meditative state, whether it was fully recognized as such or not. This state of consciousness brings a definite and blissful feeling of peace with oneself and the world. Such a moment of quietude and stillness of mind alleviates mental, emotional, and physical stress. Twenty minutes of meditation for an experienced practitioner is as restorative to the body as eight hours of sleep.

Meditation is the practice of focusing the mind and attuning to the spiritual source that lies deep within. There are many forms of meditation. Chanting sacred sounds and mantras allows one to access and integrate subtle spiritual vibrations designed for devotion, healing, and spiritual growth. Meditation and chanting with others can increase this vibratory force, bringing about powerful experiences of transcendent consciousness and life-changing miracles. One may also meditate by concentrating upon specific imagery ranging from the likeness of a saint or master to an object from nature such as a stone or sea shell.

Silent meditation, a goal in some Eastern traditions, brings the mind to a place where there is no thought, no images, and no sounds. Other philosophies encourage the transmutation of the intellectual force via methods that allow the naturally active energy field of the mind to be applied toward the attainment of better health and spiritual wisdom. Among these are the Universal Tao of China, the Alchemy of Egypt, and the Esoteric Kabbalah of the Rosicrucians.

In these traditions of Kabbalah and Alchemy, meditations based upon defined visual images are used to gather mental energy, fix it within symbolic forms, and direct this purified and refined force toward many beneficial purposes. The human capabilities of mental concentration and creative imagination are key factors in the human's ability to change existing conditions and environments. These vital powers are developed and refined by the use of alchemical meditations. The visual images that serve as the focal point in such practices are drawn from a multitude of sacred letters, words, and symbols. This is an active form of meditation that instills valuable bio-spiritual energy as well as deep relaxation.

The enlightenment traditions teach that the ability to focus, concentrate, and quiet the mind is critical to spiritual development. Yet, meditation is not the act of concentrating or quieting the mind. Meditation is best defined as a flow of consciousness that is always and endlessly in existence. By redirecting the mind inward, one is able to enter into this flow, and experience the ultimate consciousness that underlies all of manifestation. The mind can be united with and receive wisdom from this cosmic source whenever the vibrations coming in from the outer levels of consciousness are restricted. The wisdom teachings of Alchemy refer to this practice as *fixing the volatile*, a direct reference to the active nature of the outer mind that is diverted into higher expressions through meditation.

Choosing a specific focus for meditation not only develops concentration, it also stops the intrusion of unwanted thoughts and ideas. The focus may involve breath, movement, rhythmic chants, ceremony, or imagery. Such practices can help one to transcend the mind by inducing an altered state of consciousness and allowing greater spiritual energy to merge with the physical body. The practice of visualizing images and energetic movements that symbolize specific intentions is a key feature of *Alchemical Yoga*.

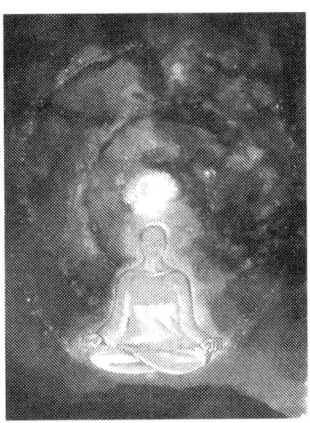

"(The Yogi) has a visible and invisible workshop. The visible one is his body, the invisible one his imagination. The imagination is a sun in the soul of man acting it its own sphere (the body), as the sun in our system acts on the earth. Wherever the sun shines, seeds planted in the soil grow, and vegetation springs up. The imagination acts in a similar manner in the soul, and calls forms of life into existence...The Spirit is the master, imagination the tool, the body the malleable material. Imagination is the power by which the will (directs) thoughts, it can (transform the body) and cure disease."
   Paracelsus

As meditation deepens, all levels of one's being are affected. The physical signs of mergence with the spirit are slow, deep breathing, a lower heart rate, and a near-suspension of bodily functions. The mind shifts from consciously creating images to witnessing a self-sustaining flow of energy. The body feels intensely alive and all emotions are transmuted into pure bliss. One who has experienced such an ecstatic state of consciousness often finds it difficult to describe it to others, as it truly transcends language.

Going within and connecting with the endless flow of consciousness is necessarily a life-changing experience. Turning away from the senses, mind, emotions, and outer world allows one to experience the self as pure, conscious, spiritual vibration. More information and greater understanding of the mysteries of the self and the universe can be obtained through proper meditation than what could be acquired through years of reading. Meditation is an inward path that leads to union with the powerful source of creation. It is the vital and life-giving stream of consciousness that creates and sustains all of existence.

Special *Alchemical Yoga* meditations have been created for use during the Living Light program. These powerful visualizations have been designed to support detoxification and speed regeneration. Exercises for increasing the powers of concentration and imagination and daily meditation practices for each week of the program are described in depth in Chapter Five.

The Sixth Key: Breath and Movement

*"Breathe long and deeply at all your meals,
that the angel of air may bless your repasts."*
The Essene Gospel of Peace.

The first act of life at birth is the inhalation of air. From that moment until the last exhale at death, the breath sustains life. Within many spiritual traditions the words used to designate the breath also mean spirit, soul, and life. In Kabbalah, the first letter of the sacred Hebrew alphabet represents the life-breath as the eternal impulse that drives universal creation.

Breathing continues automatically and unconsciously for most people, becoming unnaturally shallow over time. This unhealthy habit results in the depletion of vital life-giving oxygen in the body. Fortunately, humans have the ability to voluntarily correct the breath and improve their health.

There are a variety of breathing practices within the yogic and Kabbalistic traditions that can be used to increase oxygenation, support physical cleansing and detoxification, and aid regeneration. In addition to conscious breath work, it is critical to stimulate the heart and purify the lungs with regular invigorating exercise. Exercises such as walking, running, cycling, and swimming are excellent ways to insure sufficient oxygenation. Rebounding on a small trampoline strengthens breathing capacity and causes more oxygen to circulate throughout the body.

The science of the breath, known as *Pranayama* in the Hindu Yoga traditions, focuses on increasing oxygen intake and stimulating the metabolism in order to purify the body. Many people remain unaware of their disconnection from the endless movement of the breath in the body, allowing it to become depthless, incomplete, and rapid. Focusing one's attention on the breath while consciously inhaling deeply and exhaling fully can bring immediate relief from physical and mental tension.

When it is realized that the breath and spirit are one, it becomes possible to consider the conscious use of the breath to strengthen one's inherent spiritual energy. In Kabbalah, the soul which creates the human body as its vehicle is called *Ruach*, the word which also indicates the breath within the human form. Following the breath by placing one's attention on it as is done in breath-work leads one first into the realm of the soul, and then to *Ruach Elohim*, the creative spirit of the supernal mother.

The breath is naturally extended and balanced during physical movement, which also keeps the body fit and healthy. Establishing a regular exercise routine is an important step toward greater overall well being. Aerobic exercise is ideally done for 30 to 40 minutes three to four times a week. This type of exercise increases the heart rate and respiration, and causes one to sweat, releasing toxins through the skin.

Living Light

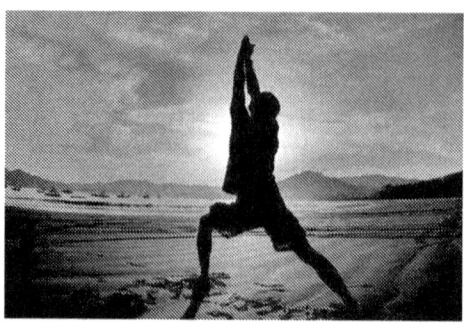

> *"Pranayama promotes the yoga principle of unification of the mind and cosmos; as we begin to transcend the distractions of mind and body, we move beyond the physical realm to far greater awareness of our inner oneness and our oneness with the universe."*
> Bri. Maya Tiwari[14]

Walking is one of the simplest and most beneficial forms of exercise. It is a completely natural human movement; however, it is undertaken by far fewer people in modern times since the advent of alternative forms of transportation. Walking can serve as a moving meditation where one consciously releases the thoughts and burdens of the day with each step. Regular walks in nature remind one of the deep connections between humanity and the earth. Whether in a city park or in the wilderness, rejuvenation takes place as one breathes deeply while walking.

Undertaking and maintaining a regular yoga practice improves breathing and instills strength and flexibility in the body. An ongoing yoga practice brings an enhanced awareness of and connection to the energetic source that fuels the body-mind organism. While providing an excellent overall workout for the body, yoga also contributes to greater mental, emotional, and spiritual harmony.

In *Alchemical Yoga*, the physical exercises of Hatha and Kundalini Yoga are combined with the visual meditations and energy movements of Alchemy. The practices also incorporate traditional breathing exercises drawn from both Eastern and Western sources. A special program of *Alchemical Yoga* practice has been created specifically for the Living Light regeneration plan and is detailed in Chapter Six.

The Seventh Key: Joy

Joy is your natural state of being. It is the bliss of the spirit manifesting through the emotional and mental bodies. This bliss is one of the greatest healing forces in the universe. If you are not experiencing it daily, find out what is blocking it from your awareness.

The mind is the creator of life's circumstances. Examine all challenges, problems, and obstacles to see the good in them. Opportunities for transformation occur daily in life. Embrace every problem as an opportunity to grow and become liberated from conditioned beliefs and emotional reactions.

Cultivating a positive mood is an important factor in health and spiritual development. Instead of predicting negative outcomes in difficult circumstances, reverse your thinking and expect miracles. Be grateful for the lessons to be learned through challenging situations. Once the lesson has been mastered, let go of the past struggle and move forward.

Every action in life offers a chance to serve as a channel for the healing love of spirit. Pass on a silent blessing to everyone you encounter. Even when you are paying the clerk in the store, you can consciously project a blessing into the money you hand over, wishing prosperity and peace for him or her. Likewise, send loving thoughts and compassion to co-workers and employers, especially those who show evidence of stress, irritation, or anger. The more positive energy you send out, the more joy you will feel.

In your daily meditation review all of the things for which you are grateful and give thanks. There is always something to be grateful for when you consider your life in relation to others in the world. I saw some of the greatest demonstrations of the healing power of gratitude when I counseled war veterans many years ago.

Those who struggled with nightmares, flashbacks, and emotional difficulties would often say, "I am grateful that all of my body is intact, some came home maimed."

One veteran who had lost an eye said, "At least I have my arms and legs, some came home without them." A man who had lost both legs and one arm said, "I am happy to be alive. Some did not come home at all." There is always room for gratitude and joy, no matter what challenges one faces in life.

Choose to spend your time with positive people, and avoid those who seem to always find fault with others and with life. You can send these down-hearted people healing love and compassion in prayer and meditation; however, when the electromagnetic fields of human bodies come into contact, a negatively charged aura will pull others downward. Focus on developing a loving fellowship with others in meditation groups, yoga classes, and spiritual gatherings.

Take time to analyze how you are spending your precious time here on earth. Are you really doing what you as a spiritual being have come here to do? Do you know what your spiritual purpose is? If not, apply all of your will and attention to finding out. Meditate on it daily, asking your higher self to reveal your true direction in life.

When you get a glimmer of your spiritual imperative, do everything in your power to manifest it in your life. Make a step-by-step plan, and take every necessary action to carry it out. This is the most important thing you can do in life. It is truly the only reason you are here. When you are doing what your spirit came here to do, your life will be filled with endless bliss. Don't wait. Do it now!

Five Ways to Turn Gloom into Joy

1. Laugh! Just start laughing, even if you have to fake it. Keep it up. In a few minutes it will become genuine. Laugh for at least ten minutes, twenty is better. Perhaps the laughter will turn to tears as tension is released. That's okay, just keep laughing. It's good for you.

2. Turn on some lively, joyous music. Get up and dance!

3. Smile! Even if you don't feel like it, make a smiley face. The muscles used in smiling will trigger a positive emotional response.

Seven Keys

4. Take a walk outdoors. As you walk, consciously release negativity. Breathe out darkness. Breathe in light. Walk for 30 minutes while meditating on turning darkness into light with each breath.

5. Close your eyes. Think of your favorite place in nature – the beach, forest, mountains – wherever you feel vibrant, happy, and alive. Visualize this place in your mind's eye. Place yourself in the picture, and get involved in the action. Feel the air, smell the scents, jump in the water, or lie in the grass. Spend several minutes on your inner vacation. Stay there until you completely believe you are there. Keep the joy of this vision with you as you slowly open your eyes.

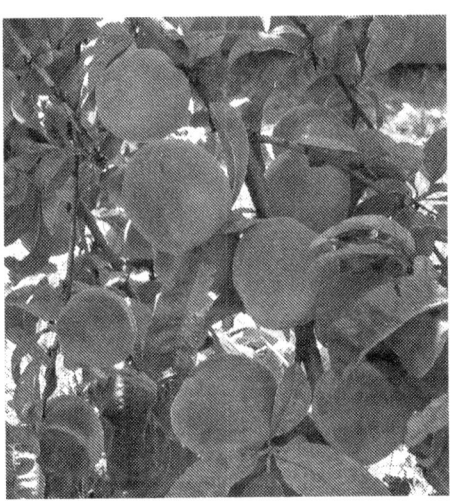

"May everyone's life be a paradise!"
Swami Muktananda[15]

How to Get the Most from the Seven Keys

1. Transition to a vegetarian diet, and work toward maintaining a diet consisting of 60-100% raw food at all times.

2. Follow the Living Light 21-day Alchemical Regeneration plan two or more times a year.

3. Fast as described in the Third Key.

4. Take plant-based digestive enzymes with all cooked foods to preserve and enhance vitality.

5. Eat super-foods for super-health and energy. Super-foods include spirulina, chlorella, wheat and barley grasses, green powder blends, sea vegetables, and bee pollen.

6. Grow and eat sprouts for increased Vital Essence.

7. Soak all seeds and nuts before consuming them to release enzyme activity.

8. Avoid sugar. Use honey, agave, or stevia for sweetness.

9. Avoid caffeine. Enjoy natural herbal teas.

10. Always buy organic produce to keep yourself, your family, and the planet healthy.

11. Eat less. Under-eating increases health and longevity.

12. Drink the water of life! Always drink fresh pure spring water whenever possible. Structured water may be an alternative, and distilled water may be used when fasting.

13. Use natural methods for healing. First seek the healing powers of whole living plants as found in a raw food diet. Discover the unique properties of living juices. The Creator gave herbs to humanity for medicine. Both fresh and dried herbs may be used to bring the body, mind, and soul into balance.

14. See a professional natural health care practitioner for specialized detoxification support, and to aid with balancing the body as needed.

15. Whenever possible, avoid prescription medicines and all synthetic drugs.

16. Acknowledge the sacred gift of food from our earthly Mother through daily prayer and conscious awareness. Before eating, visualize the plants growing in the earth, and connect spiritually with their living energy.

17. Make time to join with others in prayer, meditation, yoga, ceremony, or a sacred feast.

18. Dedicate time, energy, and attention to spiritual studies and practices, and to fulfilling the goals of your unique spiritual journey. It's the only reason you're here!

Chapter Two

Getting Ready to Regenerate

LIVING FOODS

*"The Sun is its Father; the Moon is its Mother;
the Wind carries it in its belly; its nurse is the Earth."*
The Emerald Tablet of Hermes

The Living Light 21-day Alchemical Regeneration Plan includes a diet of fruits, vegetables, sea vegetables, sprouts, grasses, juices, seeds, and dehydrated crackers, patties, and loaves. The dietary aspects of the program are designed to detoxify and rejuvenate all systems of the body. The life-renewing powers of living foods and juices increase one's physical energy and vitality, and bring greater joy and bliss into one's life. The Living Light program also supports mental and emotional cleansing, allowing the radiance of the spirit to shine through.

Superior nutrition is gained through eating whole organic fruits and vegetables in their natural raw state. Sprouted seeds, grains, legumes, and nuts are living foods that continue growing right up to the time of consumption. Raw foods contain all of the enzymes needed for the efficient digestion and assimilation of nutrition. Cooking foods at temperatures above 105°F/40°C destroys the enzymes, making it impossible to properly digest fats, proteins, and other nutrients. Heat sensitive and water-soluble vitamins and minerals are also destroyed through cooking.

The majority of one's diet should be raw fruits and vegetables, sprouted nuts, grains, and seeds. A small amount of cooked food is not harmful; however, the Living Light program is designed to cleanse and regenerate the body, and therefore does not include any cooked foods. Though nuts are live foods, with the exception of limited quantities of soaked almonds, the Living Light program does not include nuts due to their higher fat content which can delay deep cellular purification. Some delicious nut-based recipes are included in Chapter Four, and may be added to the diet following completion of the 21-day program.

Probiotics

There are a variety of microorganisms that inhabit the digestive track and help maintain proper pH levels, eliminate harmful bacteria, and stimulate the immune system. While these *probiotics* are necessary to maintain health, the various bacteria that live in the gut must be kept in careful balance. Many people suffer from an imbalance of intestinal flora as a poor diet, stress, illness, and antibiotics and other medicines destroy the good bacteria. This allows the proliferation of organisms such as Candida, a type of yeast that can produce fungal diseases when it is not controlled by the presence of helpful probiotics.

The symptoms of Candida overgrowth can mimic other disorders, and the imbalance may go undiagnosed for years as the condition worsens. If you have any of the symptoms listed below, you should consult with and follow the recommendations of your health care practitioner, and modify the Living Light diet by eliminating fruits and fruit juices, grains, legumes, and nuts.

Symptoms of Candida Overgrowth

- Digestive problems such as irritable bowel syndrome, gas, bloating, constipation, diarrhea, and intestinal cramps
- Tiredness after eating
- Craving carbohydrates (bread, pasta, pastries, etc.) and sugar

- Sensitivity to or difficulty digesting certain foods
- Rashes, itching, athletes foot, or other skin disorders
- Vaginal infections or itching
- Recurrent sinus congestion and/or sensitivity to dampness or molds in the environment
- Frequent colds, headaches, or light-headedness

The above list highlights the most common symptoms. There may be other indications that the gut has become overwhelmed with yeast. A health care practitioner can help diagnose the condition, and provide specific treatment. In general, a vegetable-based diet and sufficient intake of beneficial bacteria for a period of time can correct the problem. This diet may need to be followed for up to three months to completely restore bacterial balance.

It is also wise to avoid processed fermented foods such as beer, wine, soy sauce, and vinegars when Candida overgrowth is present. However, experiences in residential living food programs indicate that the use of fermented raw foods such as cabbage, beets, and seed cheeses can actually help to reduce Candida organisms in the body.[16] During the Living Light program it is beneficial for everyone to include extra probiotics in the diet. Probiotics can be taken in supplement form; however, fermented foods and drinks also provide a great quantity of full-spectrum friendly bacteria. Recipes for a variety of tasty fermented foods and drinks are included in Chapter Four.

Oils

Living Light recipes may include small quantities of healthy oils such as flax seed, olive, and coconut. These oils have unique nutritional value when they are used in a raw, unrefined, and unheated state. Oils should be organic and cold-pressed. Flax seed and coconut oils should be refrigerated and used within three weeks after opening. Olive oil should be stored in a dark cool place, and used within twelve weeks after opening.

Flax seed oil is a rich vegetarian source of omega-3 and omega-6 essential fatty acids. Extra-virgin olive oil is high in oleic acid, an important factor in reducing LDL (bad) cholesterol levels while increasing HDL (good) cholesterol. Olive oil is highly cleansing for the liver and gall bladder, easily digested, and high in antioxidants. Extra-virgin olive oil is recommended, as it is the least processed form. Organic, raw, unrefined, cold-pressed coconut oil is one of the healthiest foods you can consume. It is antiviral, antibacterial, and antifungal. Previously thought to be unhealthy due to its saturated fat content, coconut oil has since been found to contain medium-chain fatty acids that provide quick energy, stimulate the metabolism, and strengthen the immune system.[17]

Enzymes

Among the key elements in living foods are enzymes. Enzymes are the heart of all cellular regeneration. During digestion, enzymes transform food into the nutrients that are assimilated into the cells. Enzymes are essentially units of Vital Essence that are found within every form of life. Enzyme depletion causes aging, exhaustion, and a loss of vitality.

Enzymes carry an electromagnetic spark that fuels good health, youthfulness, and a vibrant passion for life. Cooked and processed foods contain no enzymes, and long-term, excessive consumption of such foods leads to ill health, old age, and death. This is why it is important to take supplemental plant-based enzymes with cooked foods.

Youthful cells have enzyme levels that are thousands of times greater than those found in aged cells. Young cells have a greater electrical charge than older cells, which have become dense and clogged with excess fat, protein, and environmental toxins. As these old cells lose their ability to reproduce, aging occurs. A cell that is given a source of good nutrition and regular detoxification could potentially live forever[18]

Vital Essence is at the core of every enzyme. Enzymes are the vehicles through which life renews itself within the body. High levels of metabolic enzymes within the cells are essential for the body to cleanse, heal, and regenerate. The living foods and juices used in the Living Light program provide an abundance of enzymes, which heal the digestive track and infuse dynamic energy into the cells. The result is the return of youthfulness, passion, and health.

Getting Ready to Regenerate

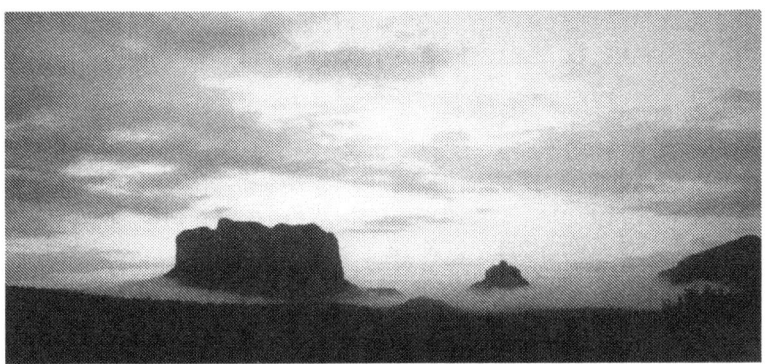

*"Seize hold of the moment before you begin
your journey to the universe within you.
However many times you falter,
seize the moment again and again."*
Gurumayi Chidvilasananda[19]

Super-Foods

The Living Light program includes super-foods such as spirulina, chlorella, wheat grass, barley grass, green powder blends, sea vegetables, and bee pollen. All of the super-foods discussed below should be stored in the refrigerator after opening to preserve their essential nutrients. Super-foods should be introduced into the diet slowly. Start with half a teaspoon of powder or half an ounce of juice daily, and increase to one to two tablespoons or ounces per day over the course of one week. Detoxification and cleansing reactions may occur when adding super-foods to the diet. Adjust your daily servings as needed.

Spirulina

Spirulina is a form of blue-green algae, believed to be the first photosynthetic life form in nature. It came into existence 3.6 billion years ago, and provided oxygenation for the evolution of all other life forms. Spirulina produces twenty times more protein per acre than soybeans. It contains a wide spectrum of nutrients including antioxidants, phytonutrients, probiotics, and nutraceuticals; all of which offer critical support to the immune system. The deep blue-green color of Spirulina gives evidence of the concentrated Vital Essence contained within this unique plant.

Chlorella

Chlorella is a single-cell, fresh water algae that is a perfect food for purification and nutrition. Chlorella binds to heavy metals, environmental poisons, and pesticide residues, and efficiently removes them from the body. It is excellent for the digestive system, and provides deep and effective colon cleansing. Chlorella also protects the liver by removing metabolic wastes, and purifying the blood.

Chlorella contains more chlorophyll per gram than any other plant. This means it will provide the highest amount of solar power. When this supercharged, congealed sunlight enters the system, the entire interior of the body is essentially flooded with light. Chlorella intensely nourishes every bodily system, and speeds regeneration by purging the blood, bowel, kidneys, and liver of the negative effects of a poor diet and toxins. Chlorella is high in vitamin D, iron, enzymes, minerals, fiber, beta-carotene, and protein. The protein found in Chlorella is superior to that contained in meat and dairy products, and provides a balanced spectrum of amino acids not found in any other natural food.

Chlorella needs to be grown organically in a pure environment, and processed in a way that preserves the vital nutrients contained in the cell wall. This type of Chlorella is known as *cracked cell wall*, the form that ensures the nutrients from within the cell are freed and may be readily assimilated into the body. Avoid Chlorella that has been freeze-dried, cooked, or pasteurized as these processes kill the essential nutrients and enzymes.

Wheat Grass

Wheat grass is an all-over tonic, blood purifier, body cleanser, and nutrient-dense food. It is the grass that Jesus spoke of in the Essene Gospel of Peace:

> *"Chew well the blades of grass as the angel of water enters our blood and gives us strength. Eat then, oh sons and daughters of Light, of this most perfect herb from the table of our Earthly Mother that your days may be long upon this earth, for such finds favor in the eyes of God."*

Wheat grass juice has a long history as a healing substance, and has been used to treat virtually every type of illness and disease. Dr. Ann Wigmore made the consumption of wheat grass popular through the healing program she established at Hippocrates Health Institute where hundreds of thousands of people have overcome numerous diseases including cancer. Wheat grass contains 20% protein, a balanced blend of twenty amino acids, iron, and twice the beta-carotene of carrots. The chemical composition of wheat grass juice closely resembles that of human red blood cells. This similarity allows its unique nutrients to be easily absorbed and synthesized by the body.

Wheat grass also holds unique spiritual powers due to the high level of chlorophyll it contains. When taken for a period of time, the juice will heal, cleanse, and balance all systems of the body. Following this purification, it can then be used alchemically to transmute the dense physical body into the body of light. Deliberate connection with the angels of the sun and earth, the spiritual guardians of the grass, and conscious absorption of its essential solar essence in the digestive track are necessary to effect this transformation.

Barley Grass

Barley grass, like wheat grass, contains an amazing spectrum of nutrients, vitamins, and minerals. Essential nutrients in barley grass include potassium, calcium, magnesium, iron, copper, phosphorus, manganese, zinc, beta-carotene, vitamins B1, B2, B6, C, and folic acid. Barley grass juice provides eleven times more calcium than milk, nearly five times more iron than spinach, and seven times more vitamin C than oranges.[20]

Homegrown, fresh, cereal grass can be juiced using a manual or electric grass juicer, or certain brands of fruit and vegetable juicers. Fresh grass juice is superior to the powdered form; however, if it is not possible for you to grow or buy grass, gently dehydrated juice powders will provide some of the essential nutrients. If you choose to grow your own grass, you will see the powerful benefits much more quickly than would be the case with dehydrated grass juice. Directions for growing grass are given below.

Super-Food Powders

Several green super-food combinations are available in powder form, and are highly beneficial when included as a regular part of one's daily diet. Super-food powders are made from whole foods; therefore, their nutritional components are more readily absorbed by the body than vitamin supplements in pill or capsule form. Quality super-food powders also contain probiotics, beneficial intestinal bacteria that can be depleted by stress, antibiotics, alcohol, and a poor diet.

Super-food powders are high in minerals, an important consideration as many people unknowingly suffer from mineral deficiencies. Super-food powders will typically include a combination of dehydrated wheat and barley grass, spirulina, chlorella, broccoli, spinach, kale, beet, alfalfa, sea vegetables, milled flax seeds, dairy-free probiotics, enzymes, and antioxidants such as green tea, bilberry, gingko biloba, and acerola berries. Avoid super-food powders that contain high quantities of fillers such as apple pectin, apple fiber, brown rice germ, and maltodextrin. Quality brands of super-food powders are listed in the Appendix.

Sea Vegetables

Sea vegetables are plants that grow deep in the ocean. They are supreme detoxifiers that offer high-powered nutition. They are available in dried form in health food stores. They contain all of the minerals found in the sea, which are the same as those found in human blood. Adding sea vegetables to the diet is an excellent way to boost mineral reserves. Sea vegetables are also high in lignans, which inhibit blood cell growth, the process by which cancer spreads in the body. They are recommended by the U.S. military to remove radioactive residues from the body following exposure, and are equally effective in eliminating heavy metals. Common sea vegetables include kelp, dulse, nori, arame, Irish moss, wakame, and kombu.

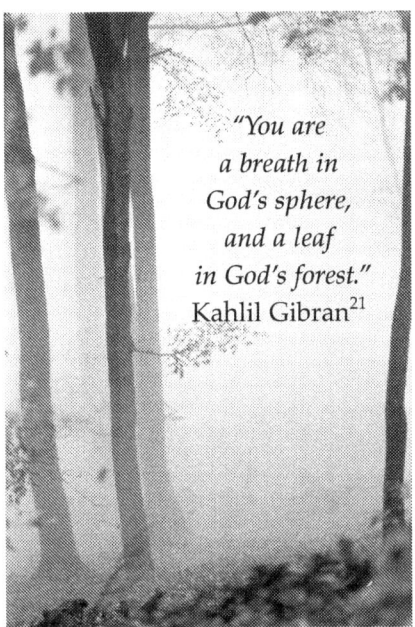

"You are
a breath in
God's sphere,
and a leaf
in God's forest."
Kahlil Gibran[21]

Bee Pollen

Bee pollen is an ancient source of nutrition that was recommended by Pythagoras for its healing abilities. Bee pollen is also extolled in the Bible, and in the sacred texts of China and Egypt. It has been referred to as nature's most complete food due to its high levels of regenerative nutrients including Rutin, B-complex, ribonucleic acid (RNA), and deoxyribonucleic acid (DNA). The bee combines pollen from deep within floral blossoms with honey from the hive. It serves as food for young bees, and contains up to 40% protein.

Bee pollen is used in many cultures throughout the world to enhance endurance and vitality, reduce cravings and addictions, protect against radiation and cancer, and overcome debilitating illnesses. It is an effective antibacterial, and increases white and red blood cells. Bee pollen has also been shown to strengthen the immune system, reduce allergic reactions, prevent the development of tumors, and increase fertility. It also stimulates the metabolism and suppresses the appetite, supporting weight loss.[22]

Bee pollen is high in enzymes and nutrient rich, and should be introduced into the diet slowly to allow the digestive system time to adapt. To test for possible allergic reactions, take one or two pollen grains at first, increasing the amount over the course of one week. The optimal amount is one tablespoon a day.

Bee pollen is a living food, and needs to be refrigerated immediately upon extraction from the hive. It should never be heated or dehydrated in processing. Avoid imported bee pollen, which is subject to over-processing and long storage. Look for quality bee pollen in the refrigerated section of health food stores.

GROWING SPROUTS

Sprouting activates the vital enzymes in nuts, seeds, legumes, and grains, making them readily available for absorption into the body. The nutritional value of nuts and seeds is greatly increased through sprouting, and the fat content is reduced by 30-40%. Sprouted foods contain high concentrations of vitamins, minerals, amino acids, protein, RNA, and DNA. This intense fusion of nutrients is only available in live cellular foods. Sprouts have a powerful regenerative effect on the body, and should be consumed daily.

Many sprouts are available ready-to-serve in supermarkets and natural food stores, but they are also very easy to grow in the kitchen at home. You will need wide-mouth glass jars covered with sprouting tops, nylon net, or cheesecloth. Be sure to purchase organic seeds whenever possible. Follow the directions below.

Small seeds such as pumpkin and sesame will be ready to harvest in one to two days. Alfalfa, fenugreek, wheat, and radish can be harvested in three to five days. Clover, buckwheat, and sunflower seeds will be ready to eat in four to five days. Begin soaking and sprouting seeds a few days before beginning the Living Light program. Place fresh sprouts in airtight containers or zip-lock bags, and store them in the refrigerator.

Sprouting Directions

1. Place the seeds in a jar, and cover it with a sprouting top or a mesh cloth secured with a rubber band.
2. Rinse with filtered water and drain through the top.
3. Cover with 3 times more pure water than seeds, and soak as specified in the chart below.
4. Drain the soak water. You can use it to water plants, but don't drink it as it may contain toxic residues. This is only an issue when sprouting seeds and nuts. Soak water from dried fruits can be used in recipes.
5. Place the jar upside down at a 45° angle in a shallow plastic container or dish drainer. The temperature in the room where the sprouts will grow should be 68-84°F /20-28°C.
6. Rinse the seeds in pure water 2 to 3 times a day, drain, and let them stand again.
7. When the sprouts reach the desired length, place them in an airtight container and store in the refrigerator.

Soak Times for Seeds, Nuts, and Fruits

Seeds	**Soak time**
Pumpkin	4 hrs
Sunflower (in hull)	8 hrs
Sesame	4 hrs
Fenugreek	6 hrs
Alfalfa	4 hrs
Flax	do not soak, grind fresh
Radish	4 hrs
Clover	6 hrs
Buckwheat	6-8 hrs
Sunflower (hulled)	4 hrs
Wheat/Barley	10-12 hrs

Nuts	**Soak time**
Almond	12 hrs
Pecan	8 hrs
Walnut	8 hrs
Macadamia	do not soak
Brazil Nuts	12 hrs
Pine Nuts	do not soak

Fruits	**Soak time**
Sun-dried tomatoes	6 hrs
Raisins, dried fruits	3-4 hrs

GROWING GREENS AND GRASSES

To grow buckwheat and sunflower greens, soak seeds in the hull, according to the chart above. Place the soaked and drained seeds just under the surface of two inches of organic soil in a planter tray with drainage holes in the bottom. Thoroughly moisten the soil with water containing powdered kelp, mixing one teaspoon of kelp with one quart of water. Cover the tray with plastic wrap and a single sheet of newspaper, and place it in a semi-dark location such as a closet (with the door open) or a basement. The shoots will grow stronger as they seek the sunlight. After three days, remove the plastic wrap and newspaper, and place the tray in the sun. Water the seedlings with kelp water as needed to keep the soil slightly damp. The greens can be harvested as soon as two leaves form and turn green. This usually takes three to five days. Store the greens in airtight containers in the refrigerator.

To grow wheat or barley grass, soak the seeds according to the chart above. Place the soaked, drained seeds on top of two inches of organic soil in a planter tray with drainage holes in the bottom. Thoroughly moisten the soil with kelp water, prepared as directed above. Cover the tray with plastic wrap and a single sheet of newspaper, and place in a semi-dark location until the grass is three inches long, which occurs in about three days. Remove the plastic wrap and paper, and place the tray in the sun. Water with kelp water as needed to keep the soil damp. The grass can be harvested when it reaches six to seven inches in length. This will usually take five to seven days.

You can leave the grass growing in the tray as you cut and juice it. Clip the grass ½ to 1 inch above the soil for juicing. Healthy grass grown in a 10" x 21" tray should produce fourteen to eighteen ounces of juice. You can allow the grass to re-grow, and harvest it a second time. After that, it must be discarded. Grass and soil remnants make great compost for the garden. Grass growing kits and juicers are available from various sources. See the Appendix for resources.

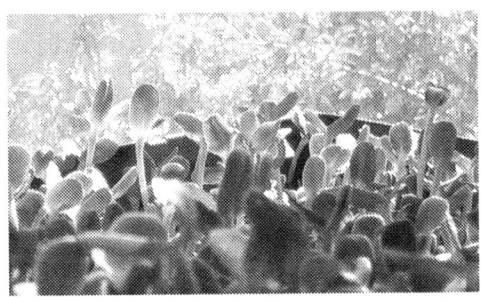

"Have they not from the time of their birth smiled in the splendor of the sun?"
P. Davidson[23]

KITCHEN EQUIPMENT

Most of the recipes in the Living Light menu plan require only sharp knives, a cutting board, and ceramic or stainless steel bowls. A few kitchen appliances are also needed. The equipment described below will make the preparation of juices and menu ingredients quick and easy.

Living Light

Blender: A blender is a basic item in the living food kitchen. It should be powerful enough to chop and liquefy raw fruits and vegetables.

Grinder: A coffee or seed grinder is an inexpensive item that can be used to mill seeds and nuts.

Juicer: The right juicer is critical for regenerating the body with living juices. A triturating juicer provides the greatest concentration of enzymes and Vital Essence. This type of juicer does not create excessive heat, and therefore preserves all of the live enzymes, fiber, minerals, and vitamins, which are the vital essence of the plant. No juice compares to the richness and intensity of juice from a triturating machine. These machines can also be used to juice wheatgrass, and produce smooth pâtés and creamy purées. For recommended juicers, see the Appendix.

Food Processor: A food processor is a versatile kitchen aid, and allows one to chop, mix, grate, or homogenize recipe ingredients instantly and effortlessly.

Dehydrator: A food dehydrator with a thermostat that can be set at or below 105° F/40° C will assist in the preparation of many alternative food items in living food recipes such as crackers, patties, and loaves.

BUYING AND PREPARING FOOD

Organic foods offer superior nutrition without the health hazards that come from chemical farming and genetically modified organisms (GMO's). Organic farming aids the production of quality food while maintaining the ecological balance of the earth. Organic foods contain higher amounts of essential vitamins, minerals, and antioxidants than conventionally produced foods.

To preserve your health at all times, and to receive the greatest benefits from the Living Light program, you should purchase only organically grown fruits, vegetables, nuts, seeds, and grains. If some recipe ingredients are not available in organic form, consider replacing them with other organic items.

It may sometimes be necessary to use conventionally grown foods where organic supplies are not available. Non-organic produce contains smaller amounts of chemical residues than do meat and dairy products. The body can cleanse itself following minor exposure to pesticides, especially when following the Living Light program. Do your best to take care of your body, and purchase fresh, organic, raw foods from whole food supermarkets, health stores, and farmer's markets whenever possible. Below is a list of key ingredients to help you get ready to regenerate.

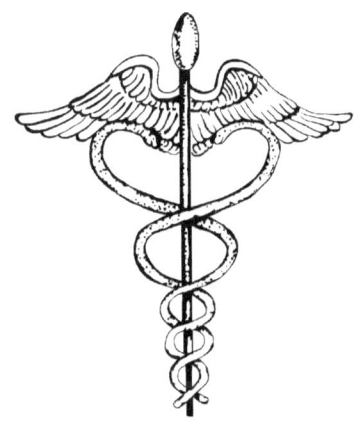

*"Man eats solar vibrations trapped in nutrients.
Enzymes, proteins, vitamins are temporary
energy traps; under the action of enzymes in
the body, energies are released for building
and maintenance of the human body.
Some individuals get the necessary
nutrients via sun and color;
most via food."*
Viktoras Kulvinskas[24]

Living Light Shopping List

Vegetables
Lettuce
Carrots
Celery
Tomatoes
Spinach
Cucumbers
Beets
Parsley
Bell Peppers
Kale
Green Onions
Zucchini
Broccoli
Cauliflower
Spaghetti Squash
Cabbage
Corn
Yellow Squash
Eggplant
Mushrooms
Shallots
Ginger Root
Garlic
Radishes
Watercress

Fruits
Apples
Bananas
Pears
Melons
Peaches
Avocados
Lemons
Berries
Papaya
Pineapple
Mango
Limes
Grapefruit
Dates
Oranges
Figs
Apricots
Cherries
Plums
Grapes
Olives
Raisins
Coconut
Kiwi Fruit
Sun Dried Tomatoes

Seed/Nuts
Almonds
Sunflower
Pumpkin
Sesame
Clover
Flax
Broccoli
Radish
Fenugreek
Alfalfa
Hemp

Oils
Flax Seed
Olive
Coconut
Hemp

Living Light Shopping List

Super-foods
Spirulina
Chlorella
Green Powder
Bee Pollen
Dehydrated Wheat Gras
Dehydrated Barley Grass

Grains
Wheat
Buckwheat
Rye
Quinoa
Millet

Legumes for Sprouting
Chick Peas
Mung Beans
Lentils

Other Items
Mineral/Sea Salt
Black Pepper
Raw Apple Cider Vinegar
Fresh/Dried Herbs
Herbal Teas
Spices
Dried Sea Vegetables
Raw Chocolate/Carob

Fresh raw foods form the basis of an interesting and delicious diet when they are prepared and offered in a variety of shapes and textures. In addition to slicing, dicing, shredding, and grating, vegetables and fruits can also be puréed using a food processor, high-speed blender, or quality juicer. Avoid boring salads and keep your taste buds happy by chopping green leaves into bite-sized pieces, and cutting ingredients into cubes, rounds, and other interesting shapes. A spiral slicer is great for creating vegetable noodles and pastas, and a mandoline uniformly slices vegetables and fruits thick or thin, and easily juliennes, grates, and shreds. Resources for helpful kitchen equipment can be found in the Appendix.

Begin sprouting, growing grasses and greens, and dehydrating foods one week before beginning the Living Light program. Organize a sprouting, growing, and dehydration schedule to be sure you will have fresh greens, sprouts, crackers, and breads as needed. Pure water is also a critical component in regeneration, and a reliable source for spring, purified, or distilled water should be established before you begin the program.

Cleansing From The Inside Out

The Living Light plan is designed to help cleanse the body of toxins, wastes, and impurities. The program incorporates raw foods and juices, super-foods, herbal teas, meditation, yoga, and internal cleansing via enemas or colon hydrotherapy. As super-nutritious raw foods enter the body, the effects of many years of poor dietary habits, stress, and environmental contamination are eradicated.

As toxins break free from the cells, organs, muscles, and fat stores of the body, they must be removed through the kidneys, skin, lungs, and colon. For most people this process can result in an overload of these eliminative systems. The debris from intense cleansing can become trapped in the colon, leading to a re-absorption of the poisons they contain. The best way to reduce or avoid unpleasant cleansing reactions such as nausea, headaches, fatigue, and body aches is to support the process of elimination with herbal

Getting Ready to Regenerate

laxatives, regular enemas, or colon hydrotherapy.

Herbal laxative teas and infusions can provide important support for the cleansing process by assisting the colon to thoroughly remove toxic debris. Effective herbal ingredients include cascara sagrada bark, rhubarb root, licorice root, buckthorn, and slippery elm. Quality herbal colon cleansing kits work very well in conjunction with the Living Light program, and are highly recommended. These products contain a combination of cleansing herbs in capsule form. Resources for recommended supplements that aid colon cleansing can be found in the Appendix.

For centuries a basic component of health recovery has been the administration of enemas. Modern medicine has shifted away from this healing protocol with dreadful consequences. An enema is one of the least expensive and most beneficial therapies that one can undertake at home. With the introduction of modern colon hydrotherapy equipment, professional colonic treatments offer a great advantage over self-administered enemas. A colonic introduces water into the colon using medically approved devices and disposable speculums. After a time the water is expelled, and the colon is filled again. This process may be repeated several times during a colonics session.

It is useful to begin with self-administered enemas daily or every other day for the first week of the Living Light program. For the remaining two weeks, enemas may be taken once or twice a week. This will ensure that toxins are thoroughly removed from the body as they are being purged from the cells. Some people are averse to enemas due to embarrassment, negative past experiences, or a lack of information. In beginning the Living Light program, you are taking positive steps to restore health and bring greater radiance into your life. Keep an open mind about internal cleansing, and give it a try. Those who have done so report feeling lighter and happier as a consequence.

You may prefer to receive professional colon hydrotherapy in place of self-administered enemas. Colonics are more effective, and should be undertaken once or twice each week of the Living Light program, and once during the week following completion. Consult with a colonic therapist in your area to work out a plan that best suits your needs. Certified practitioners are listed with the

International Association for Colon Hydrotherapy. See the Appendix for contact information and other resources.

Enema Procedure

1. Connect the enema bag with the enema tube, and the enema tube with the enema nozzle.
2. Fill the enema bag with one half to one liter of filtered or distilled water at body temperature.
3. Clamp the enema tube.
4. Hang the enema bag about three to four feet above the floor.
5. Lie on your back on the floor.
6. Lubricate your anus and the enema nozzle with olive oil.
7. Slowly and gently insert the nozzle into your anus.
8. Release the clamp. The enema liquid will flow into the lower colon.
9. Clamp the tubing as soon as you feel a sensation of fullness, or when the bag is empty.
10. Remove the nozzle from your anus.
11. Turn so that you are lying on your left side. If possible, without forcing yourself, retain the enema for two to ten minutes while lying down and massaging your abdomen.
12. Empty your bowel.
13. After emptying your bowel, you can repeat the process until the bag is empty.

To maintain the balance of electrolytes during times of frequent enema use, add one teaspoon of baking soda. Enema bags and kits are available at pharmacies and health stores as well as through the Internet.

Getting Ready to Regenerate

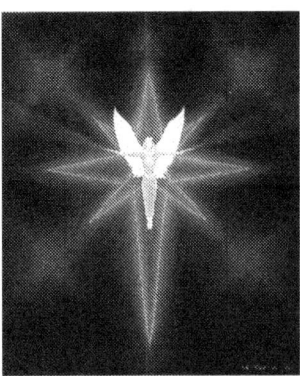

*"Think not that it is sufficient that the
angel of water embrace you outwards only.
I tell you truly, baptism with water
frees you from all disease."*
The Gospel of Peace[25]

SUPPORT FOR BODY, MIND, AND SOUL

The Living Light program incorporates a diet of 100% living foods and fresh juices in order to purify and regenerate the physical body. However, the consumption of these foods is only one component of the program, which is designed to bring about greater health and increased spiritual clarity. Changing the cellular consciousness of the body is significantly aided through the use of specialized alchemical meditations. These meditations use visualizations that activate and increase Vital Essence.

What is held in mind consistently will ultimately manifest as a tangible physical reality. The mind and emotions not only create the physical body, they also bring about all of the circumstances in one's life. Often this process operates unconsciously, introducing undesirable consequences into one's environment. It is also a primary source of stress, strain, and toxic conditions in the body. By working with the alchemical meditations detailed in Chapter Five, a new pattern is created, which the regenerated cells may follow to rebuild the body.

Living Light

Yoga, breath-work, and exercise also speed the process of rejuvenation, aiding the body to throw off toxic debris. Yoga offers excellent support for the whole person as it incorporates deep breathing and stretching, and quiets the mind. Certain *Alchemical Yoga* postures and practices have been selected for use during the Living Light program, and are explained in depth in Chapter Six.

Designating a special place in your home for meditation and yoga helps develop self-discipline, and creates a space in which the higher energies produced by the practices can build up over time. Meditation does not require a large space, a small table arranged as a healing altar can be placed in one's bedroom or any corner. Yoga practice requires enough room to lie down and stretch out fully.

As you proceed through the Living Light program it can be beneficial to receive massage therapy, which helps the body process and eliminate toxins. Chiropractic adjustments can also help the body to regain its proper balance. Regular sessions in a steam room and/or dry sauna allow the skin to cleanse as it sweats out poisons. Steam baths and saunas also increase circulation, relax the muscles, and stimulate the immune system. A detoxification bath may be created at home by adding Epsom salts to very warm water, and soaking in it for up to one hour.

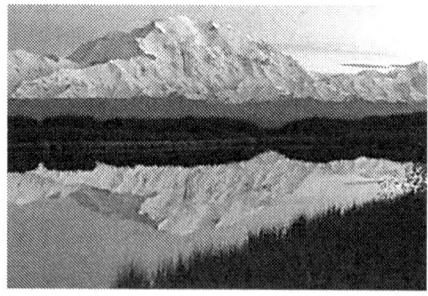

"You may make Heaven descend
upon Earth, so that it may abide in you."
Jesus, The Book of Knowledge of the Invisible[26]

Chapter Three

The Living Light Program

PREPARATION WEEK

*"In the beginning, he decided to have his
likeness become a great power."*
The Sophia of Jesus Christ[27]

The Living Light plan begins with a one-week transitional diet that prepares the body to receive all of the benefits of the twenty-one days that follow. This first step involves simple modifications to your usual diet, and an introductory daily meditation that stimulates cleansing while attuning the body and mind to the process of regeneration. During this week, raw foods form 50% of the diet, which gently starts the process of digestive clearing. Dense protein foods such as meat, dairy, and soy, and all processed foods are eliminated from the diet at this time. Coffee, caffeine, and alcohol are gradually reduced and then removed.

    The preparation week is important in several ways. It eases the transition from a cooked food diet to a 100% living food diet. Throughout this week, your body will begin to adjust to a greater intake of raw foods. Adding 50% raw foods to the diet will initiate liver and colon cleansing, reducing the severity of unpleasant cleansing reactions once the full program is begun. The transition period also allows you to become familiar with the preparation of living foods, and to learn a few of the Living Light program recipes. Preparation week is a good time to gather supplies, begin growing greens and grasses, and make dehydrated foods.

While the preparation week is especially critical for those whose present diet includes meat, it is also important for vegetarians who consume dairy, processed foods, and soy products, and for vegans whose diet contains processed foods and soy. Meat, dairy, and soy are eliminated from the diet during the preparation week as they delay digestion and carry potential health risks. The average Western diet contains far too much protein from meat and dairy products, which often results in serious health problems. Excessive protein intake can cause kidney disease, cancers, cardiovascular disease, and osteoporosis as well as other disorders.[28]

The idea that sufficient protein can only be obtained with a diet that includes meat, dairy, and soy is a myth. Plant foods contain ample amounts of protein and amino acids. This can be seen clearly in the animal kingdom where large, powerful, healthy animals consume only living plants. Even the animals that are consumed for meat are natural vegetarians.

Although soy is derived from a plant, it is most commonly consumed in heavily processed forms such as tofu, tempeh, and vegetarian meat substitutes, which have been linked to health and reproductive problems. Soybeans were traditionally fermented for long periods of time to produce tofu. Now tofu is mass-produced in factories in a process that does not completely remove the naturally occurring toxins found in soy, and which may also introduce undesirable chemical changes.[29] Living Light recipes include only small amounts of fermented soy in the form of tamari sauce and miso.

During preparation week other processed foods are also avoided. These foods include refined sugar, salt, and wheat, snack foods, soft drinks, and canned, packaged, and frozen foods. Such foods have no real nutritional value, cause many health problems, and burden the digestive system due to their lack of enzymes. Eliminating these foods prior to beginning the 21-day Living Light program initiates the process of cleansing from the effects of such foods, and allows the digestive track to improve its absorption of essential nutrients.

Coffee, alcohol, and caffeine drinks need to be reduced and then eliminated during the preparation week. This allows the body to gradually detoxify from these substances, and reduces the severity of headaches and other symptoms associated with withdrawal. If one's diet includes caffeine drinks and/or alcohol on a daily basis, these items are incrementally reduced over the first four days of the preparation week. For example, if you typically drink one cup of coffee daily, have only ¾ cup on day one of preparation week. On day two, drink ½ cup. Decrease consumption to ¼ cup on day three, ⅛ cup on day four, and have no coffee on day five. This method can be used for any caffeinated or alcoholic drinks.

The preparation week diet includes 50% healthy cooked foods and 50% raw foods. Foods to eat or avoid are listed below, along with a sample daily menu plan. Additional 50/50 menus can be created using the recipes in Chapter Four. If one's diet does not presently include meat, dairy, soy, processed foods, caffeine drinks, or alcohol, and already incorporates a minimum of 50% raw foods, the preparation week diet is not needed. In this case, simply begin daily practice of the preparation week meditation as described below.

In addition to dietary modifications, the preparation week alchemical meditation, *Purifying Light*, should be practiced daily for one week before beginning the Living Light program. *Purifying Light* lays the foundation for all of the other alchemical meditations used during each week of the program. All of the Living Light meditations are described in detail in Chapter Five.

Preparation Week Diet

Foods to Eat

All fresh fruits
All vegetables, raw or cooked
All sprouts
All nuts, fresh coconut,
  and nut milks
All seeds and seed milks
Dried fruits
Whole grains and legumes
Mineral or sea salt
Fresh or dried seasoning herbs
Raw, organic olive, flax, coconut oils
Fresh fruit and vegetable juices
Super-food powders
Sea vegetables
Raw apple cider vinegar
Wheat grass juice
Herbal teas
Honey, Stevia

Foods to Avoid

Refined sugar
Refined wheat breads
Sweet snacks and candy
Beef, pork, poultry, fish
Soft drinks
Fried foods
Processed foods
Refined salt
Soy products
Vegetable and animal oils
Caffeine and alcohol
Milk, butter, eggs, and
  all dairy products
Canned and frozen foods
Distilled vinegar
Packaged and
  preserved foods
Artificial sweeteners

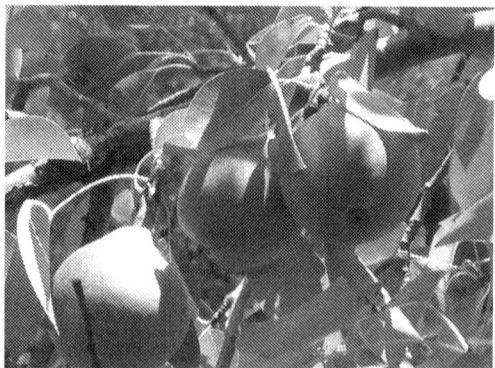

*"Daniel said, 'Give us vegetables to eat and
water to drink. Then see how we look...'
After ten days they looked healthier and better
than any of the young men who ate at the royal table."*
The Book of Daniel, Chapter One, Verses 11-15

Preparation Week Sample Daily Menu

Breakfast:

Fresh Fruit Juice
Herbal Tea
Morning Granola* with Almond Milk*
Banana Coconut Smoothie*

Lunch:

Fresh Vegetable Juice
Garden Salad* with Tomato Basil Dressing*
Steamed Mixed Squash with Millet

Dinner:

Spinach Caesar Salad*
Baked Potato with Flax Oil and Parsley
Apple Nutmeg Delight*

Snack Choices:

Fresh Fruit
Sliced Vegetables with Guacamole Dip*
Banana Coconut Smoothie*
Super Green Smoothie*
Flax Crackers*
Dried Fruits and Soaked Nuts

*See Chapter Four for recipes

LIVING LIGHT

The Living Light program centers on a 100% living food diet, fresh juices, and super-foods in conjunction with key alchemical mediations and yoga practices. Internal cleansing using enemas or colonics and herbal laxative teas or supplements enhance the program's effectiveness. The Living Light diet provides superior nutrition and enables the body to experience a deep purification process that leads to cellular regeneration. Living Light is a holistic program, offering healing, nourishment, and balance for the body, mind, and soul.

The Living Light program is beneficial for virtually everyone; however, you should consult a health care professional to assess your health status before undertaking any new exercise or diet program. Those with diabetes or other sugar-related imbalances will benefit by eliminating fruits, carrots, beets, and other high sugar foods from the program. Certain medications may need to be adjusted as more fresh living foods are consumed. Be sure to consult with and follow the advice of your health care provider before and during the program if you are taking any prescription medicines or have special health conditions.

The three-week Living Light program offers a unique opportunity to experience the many benefits that come from eating food in its natural state. Once the remnants of dense cooked foods have cleared from the body, the pure nutrition of fresh organic produce and juices is rapidly absorbed into the cells, blood, and organs. The rewards to be gained through the program include increased physical energy, weight loss, mental clarity, and a feeling of blissful peace and contentment. These are signs that the Vital Essence is returning and increasing, and the body is taking on more light.

The daily menu plans include an abundance of health-giving foods presented in a variety of rich and tasty dishes. Nourishing juices, delectable smoothies, and heavenly raw treats offer high-energy snacks and desserts. Special daily meditations soothe the mind and guide the body to heal, repair, and rejuvenate. Living Light yoga practices focus on strengthening the eliminative systems to aid detoxification while providing deep relaxation and stress relief.

During the first week of the program the pH balance in the body will become more alkaline. This is an important adjustment as an overly acidic physiological environment is the root condition that allows the disease process to begin. A correct pH balance must be maintained within the body in order for the cells to remain energized and healthy. Eating meats, dairy, caffeine, alcohol, processed and cooked foods increases acidity, while fresh raw fruits, vegetables, grasses, and super-foods increase alkalinity. Key factors that contribute to the alkalizing power of plants are their abundance of enzymes and organic minerals.

Acidity in the body also increases due to mental stress, negative emotional states, improper breathing, and environmental toxins. The Living Light plan increases alkalinity with a raw food diet and juices while the alchemical meditations relieve acidic mental and emotional conditions. Daily yoga practice also helps to balance the body's pH by increasing oxygenation, stimulating detoxification, and alleviating the physical effects of stress.

As the bodily systems become more alkaline, deep cleansing occurs. Old stores of toxins and partially digested food remnants begin to break free and are released through the eliminative systems of the kidneys, lungs, skin, and colon. During the first week of the program, one may experience mild to moderate cleansing reactions such as headaches, nausea, constipation, bad breath, fatigue, and chills. These symptoms occur when the toxic matter begins to circulate in the blood stream, placing a heavy load upon the body's natural decontamination processes.

It is vital during this time to maintain supportive measures such as consuming herbal laxative teas or supplements, and undertaking daily enemas or colonics once or twice a week. If one is experiencing two to three bowel movements daily, colonic cleansing support may not be needed. If diarrhea occurs these methods should be avoided; and if it persists one should seek advice from a health care professional.

In the second week of the program, the built up debris will be moving out of the body more freely, and the pH balance will begin a definite shift into higher alkalinity. The physical effects of this alkaline increase include improvements to the digestive track, liver, blood supply, kidneys, and other vital organs. One will typically experience increased energy, a clearer mind, and an elevated mood. These are the initial signs that the cells of the body are healing, purifying, and taking in more light.

By the third week, the cells and organs of the body will be well into the regenerating process. States of bliss, great physical well-being, and extraordinary mental sharpness are among the many benefits that may be experienced in the last week of the program. One's appearance may become quite radiant, and the body generally feels much lighter. Much internal contamination will have cleared by this time, and the cellular system will be rapidly regenerating. Youthfulness, high energy, and happiness predominate as Vital Essence accumulates and spreads throughout the body.

Each week of the Living Light Program includes a one-day juice fast. This fasting day allows the digestive system to rest, speeds detoxification, and also provides an opportunity for one to relax, meditate, and reflect on one's goals and progress. During each fasting day, fresh organic juices are consumed along with plenty of pure water, herbal teas, and a special vegetable broth that aids the cleansing process. The alchemical meditation, *Fountain of Sustenance*, which transmutes solar energy into physical nutrition, is performed on this day. This meditation is described in Chapter Five, which includes all of the Living Light program meditations.

Each fasting day ideally should be set aside as a day to rest, study, and meditate. Avoid visitors, television, newspapers, the Internet, and radio programs during this day. Focus on soothing the body, mind, and soul by reading inspirational materials and books, listening to uplifting music and sacred chants, soaking in a hot bath, or enjoying a quiet walk in nature. This day is a good time to indulge in an afternoon nap, a relaxing massage, and writing in a journal or diary. The fasting day serves as the transition point from one week of the program to the next, marking your steady progress toward better health, greater peace, and increased happiness.

LIVING LIGHT SAMPLE WEEKLY MENUS

A wide variety of menu choices are available during the Living Light program, offering superb nutrition and fabulous meals. The sample menus below provide a complete balanced diet, and contain all of the elements needed for a healthy energetic life. The meals are easy to digest, providing an abundance of enzymes, minerals, vitamins, and amino acids.

Each day begins with a *Morning Elixir* of wheat grass juice or a super-food drink consumed after yoga or exercise. Breakfast may be eaten one hour after the Elixir. One additional serving of wheat grass juice may be taken between lunch and dinner. Additional super-food powder drinks can be taken anytime throughout the day.

Chapter Four contains all of the recipes for the meals listed in the sample menus along with many others that will inspire, entice, and satisfy. Use the sample menus only as a guide to get started. Be creative and add your own unique touches to the recipes, or create a completely new raw meal based on a favorite cooked dish. Review and organize recipe ingredients that may require advance preparation such as fermented and dehydrated foods, grasses, and sprouts. Experiment, create, and enjoy!

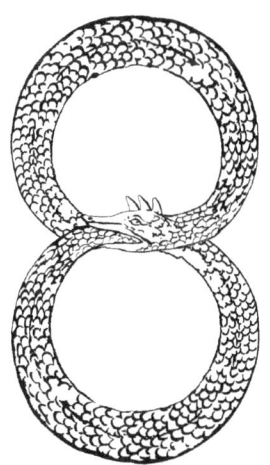

Living Light

Menu Plan for Sunday

Morning Elixir:

1 oz. fresh Wheat Grass Juice
or
1 T Super-food Powder in 6 oz. Juice or Water

Breakfast:

Fresh Fruits with Super Seed Mix
Essene Bread with Raw Honey
Fresh Apple Juice
Herbal Tea

Lunch:

Raw Tacos
Sprout Salad with Creamy Cilantro Dressing
Fresh Vegetable Juice
Herbal Tea

Dinner:

Greek Salad with Seed Cheese
Creamy Tomato Soup
Flax Crackers
Herbal Tea

The Living Light Program

Menu Plan for Monday

Morning Elixir:

1 oz. fresh Wheat Grass Juice
or
1 T Super-food Powder in 6 oz. Juice or Water

Breakfast:

Dried Fruit and Seed Granola
Berry Fruigurt
Fresh Fruit Juice
Herbal Tea

Lunch:

Ocean Salad with Tamari Dressing
Nori Crackers
Fresh Vegetable Juice
Herbal Tea

Dinner:

Vegetable Loaf
Creamy Sweet Potatoes
Garden Salad with Tangy Tomato Dressing
Herbal Tea

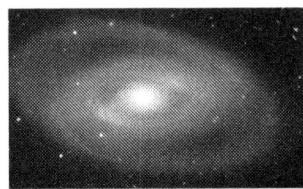

*"Every living thing breathes and intakes this
Light freely, and to none is it exclusive or private."*
Israel Regardie[30]

Menu Plan for Tuesday

Morning Elixir:

1 oz. fresh Wheat Grass Juice
or
1 T Super-food Powder in 6 oz. Juice or Water

Breakfast:

Super Green Smoothie
Essene Bread with Raw Raspberry Jam
Fresh Fruit Juice
Herbal Tea

Lunch:

Falafel with Raw Hummus
Cucumber Dill Salad
Fresh Vegetable Juice
Herbal Tea

Dinner:

Garden Salad with Italian Dressing
Spaghetti Squash with Zesty Marinara Sauce
Garlic Seed Bread
Herbal Tea

Menu Plan for Wednesday

Morning Elixir:

1 oz. fresh Wheat Grass Juice
or
1 T Super-food Powder in 6 oz. Juice or Water

Breakfast:

Wheat Berry Porridge
Orange Banana Fruigurt
Fresh Fruit Juice
Herbal Tea

Lunch:

Tabouli
Tomato Basil Salad with Mixed Greens
Turkish Flat Bread
Fresh Vegetable Juice
Herbal Tea

Dinner:

Sun Burgers
California Coleslaw
Beet Relish and Crispy Pickles
Herbal Tea

Living Light

Menu Plan for Thursday

Morning Elixir:

1 oz. fresh Wheat Grass Juice
or
1 T Super-food Powder in 6 oz. Juice or Water

Breakfast:

Morning Granola with Almond Milk
Fresh Fruit Juice
Herbal Tea

Lunch:

Broccoli and Apple Salad
Flax Crackers with Avocado Dip
Fresh Vegetable Juice
Herbal Tea

Dinner:

Extraordinary Mushroom Pâté
Sesame Kale Salad
Antipasto Treats
Herbal Tea

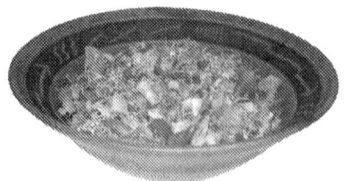

"As we cleanse and purify our bodies
we develop a keen sense of what is
healthiest and best for us to eat."
Paul Bragg[31]

Menu Plan for Friday

Morning Elixir:

1 oz. fresh Wheat Grass Juice
or
1 T Super-food Powder in 6 oz. Juice or Water

Breakfast:

Diced Apples & Raisins with Super Seed Mix
Banana Coconut Fruigurt
Fresh Fruit Juice
Herbal Tea

Lunch:

Tossed Chinese Vegetables
Sushi Rolls
Miso Soup
Fresh Vegetable Juice

Dinner:

Basil Bean Salad
Almond Seed Pâté
Sprout Salad with Avonaise
Herbal Tea

Menu Plan for Saturday

Juice Fasting Day

Morning Elixir:

1 oz. fresh Wheat Grass Juice
or
1 T Super-food Powder in 6 oz. Juice or Water

Breakfast:

Apple Pear Juice

Mid-Morning:

Mineral Magic Juice

Lunch:

Alkalizing Broth

Mid-Afternoon:

Mega-Green Juice

Dinner:

Super Seven Juice

"You see – meditation happens, understanding happens, acceptance happens, surrender happens. And when that happens, you know it – because there is a feeling of emptiness."
Ramesh Balsekar[32]

LIVING LIGHT SAMPLE DAILY SCHEDULES

Day One

6:00 AM:
Alchemical Meditation

6:45 AM:
Alchemical Yoga Practices

7:30 AM:
Morning Elixir

8:30 AM:
Breakfast

12:30 PM:
Lunch

5:30 PM:
Walk in Nature

6:15 PM:
Dinner

7:30 PM:
Alchemical Meditation

Day Two

6:00 AM:
Alchemical Meditation

6:45 AM:
Aerobic Exercise

7:30 AM:
Morning Elixir

8:30 AM:
Breakfast

12:30 PM:
Lunch

5:30 PM:
Alchemical Yoga Practices

6:15 PM:
Dinner

7:30 PM:
Alchemical Meditation

All of the important components of the Living Light program can easily be incorporated into your daily life. The ideal schedule for each week of the program includes the Living Light meditations and yoga practices on a daily basis, and aerobic exercise and brisk walking at least three times per week. This ideal can be accomplished by alternating use of the Day One and Day Two schedules in the sample above.

AFTER THE PROGRAM

Following completion of the Living Light program, one may return to the inclusion of cooked foods in the diet if desired. For the first week, cooked items should be limited to steamed or baked vegetables, and should form no more than 20% of the diet. Cooked whole grain foods may be gradually reintroduced the following week.

Returning to a diet that includes meat is not recommended as this will quickly reverse the gains that have been made during the program. If your diet included meat before the program, consider consolidating your progress by maintaining a vegetarian diet. If you choose to include meat in your diet, please do so infrequently, in small amounts, and in strictly organic forms.

This is also a good time to do away with processed foods that have no nutritional value. Dairy and soy may be included occasionally; however, keep in mind that these items can contribute to undesirable physical effects if they form more than a small percentage of the diet. Raw dairy products that contain the enzymes needed for digestion are preferred over pasteurized milk, cheeses, and yogurt that are subjected to heat and difficult to digest.

In the weeks that follow the program, work to maintain a diet that includes 60 to 100% raw foods. This will allow you to sustain the benefits received from the program, and will contribute to greater health and well-being. Continued daily use of super-foods and a weekly one-day juice fast will keep the body energized and oriented toward further regeneration. One will also benefit greatly from continued practice of the alchemical meditations, yoga, and regular exercise.

An 80 to 100% raw food diet can be maintained for life, and will bring numerous health benefits while continuing to slow the aging process by stimulating cellular regeneration. Living Light can serve as a complete dietary program that supports a high energy lifestyle with supreme nutrition and delicious foods. If less desirable foods once again become a substantial part of the diet, the Living Light program may be repeated as often as desired. The program is ideal for regular detoxification and rejuvenation, and should be undertaken two or more times a year for best results. Chapter Seven contains additional information to help you continue to thrive beyond Living Light.

Chapter Four

Living Light Recipes

SAUCES, DIPS, SPREADS, AND DRESSINGS

Avonaise

½ avocado
¼ C ground pumpkin
  & sunflower seeds
½ garlic clove
Mineral or sea salt to taste
Fresh ground black pepper
1 t celery seeds, rubbed
4-5 T raw apple cider vinegar
Water

Place avocado, ground seeds, garlic, salt, pepper, and celery seeds in a blender. Add apple cider vinegar and process until creamy. Add water 1 tablespoon at a time as needed to create a thick and creamy mixture. Use as a dressing for coleslaw and salads, or as a spread or dip.

Living Light

Raw Hummus

2 C sprouted chickpeas
   or soaked almonds
3 T raw Tahini
½ clove garlic
Juice of two lemons
Mineral or sea salt to taste

Blend all ingredients in a food processor or blender, adding water as needed to produce a smooth and thick consistency. Optional variations include adding diced, soaked sun-dried tomatoes, ¼ t cayenne pepper, or ¼ t curry powder.

Cranberry Sauce

1¼ C fresh cranberries
1 orange, peeled
1 t orange zest
Four to six dates

Blend cranberries and orange in a blender or food processor, leaving the mixture chunky. Add four dates and zest, taste and add more dates as desired to make the mixture tangy-sweet. Place in a covered dish and refrigerate before serving.

Raw Raspberry Jam

½ C fresh raspberries
1 t lemon juice
1 T raw honey or a pinch
   of stevia

Place all ingredients in a blender or food processor and purée. Serve immediately or store in the refrigerator.

Zesty Marinara Sauce

2 zucchinis cut into bite-sized slivers
½ C sliced black olives
¼ C soaked sun-dried tomatoes
1 shallot
½ clove garlic
2 medium tomatoes
½ t dried oregano
1 t dried basil, or ¼ C fresh basil, minced
Fresh ground black pepper
Mineral or sea salt to taste

Roughly chop half of the sun-dried tomatoes and place in a medium bowl with the zucchini pieces and black olives. Blend remaining ingredients in a food processor or blender, until the mixture forms a thick sauce. Add the sauce to zucchini mix, and stir well. Serve immediately, or store in refrigerator overnight. Serve over grated spaghetti squash or use in *Live Lasagna* or *Raw Pizza*.

Spicy Mexican Salsa

3 tomatoes
½ clove garlic
½ medium onion
¼ C fresh cilantro
1-4 fresh jalapeno peppers, quartered and seeded
Mineral or sea salt to taste

Pulse-process all ingredients in a food processor or blender to desired consistency. Use only as much jalapeno pepper as tolerated.

Bean and Corn Salsa

1 C sprouted mung beans
Corn removed from 1 fresh cob
1 tomato, diced
1 avocado, diced
1 shallot, minced
¼ C fresh cilantro, roughly chopped
¼ t chili powder
Mineral or sea salt to taste
Juice of one lime

Place all vegetables and seasonings in a medium bowl, squeeze lime juice over all, and mix well. Serve immediately or refrigerate for up to one hour.

Guacamole Dip

1 large avocado, quartered
1 medium tomato, chopped
2 green onions, chopped
¼ C cilantro, chopped
¼ t chili powder
Mineral or sea salt to taste
Juice of one lime

Place avocado pieces in a bowl. Mash the avocado with a fork, leaving a few small chunks. Add all other ingredients, and stir gently. Serve immediately.

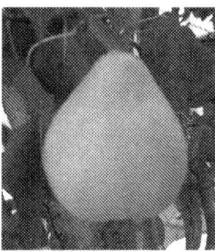

"Love and let love. Rejoice in every shape of love, and get thy rapture and thy nourishment thereof."
The Master Therion[33]

Creamy Cilantro Dressing

1 avocado
1 C cilantro leaves
¼ C olive oil
3 T apple cider vinegar
Mineral or sea salt to taste

Blend avocado, cilantro leaves, and olive oil in a blender or food processor until smooth. Add remaining ingredients and process until creamy.

Tamari Dressing

¼ C flax oil
3 T apple cider vinegar
3 T wheat-free tamari sauce
3 T orange juice

Whisk all ingredients together, and store in the refrigerator in a glass bottle or jar. Shake well before serving.

Tangy Tomato Dressing

3 tomatoes
5-6 soaked sun-dried tomatoes
1 small red bell pepper
1 shallot
½ clove garlic
⅛ C ground sunflower seeds
3 T fresh basil
3 T lemon juice
¼ C olive oil
¼ t dried crushed
   red pepper, optional

Place fresh and sun-dried tomatoes, lemon juice, and olive oil in a blender or food processor and blend until smooth. Add remaining ingredients and process until well blended. Store in refrigerator and shake well before serving.

Tomato Basil Dressing

3 tomatoes
⅛ C fresh basil
¼ C flax oil
3 T apple cider vinegar
Fresh ground black pepper
Mineral or sea salt to taste

Process all ingredients in a food processor or blender until liquefied. Store in refrigerator and shake well before serving.

Italian Dressing

½ C olive oil
4 T apple cider vinegar
1 T lemon juice
2 t minced fresh parsley
   or 1 t dried parsley
2 t minced fresh basil
   or 1 t dried basil
1½ t minced fresh oregano
   or ¼ t dried oregano
½ t minced fresh thyme
   or ¼ t dried thyme
¼ t fresh ground black pepper
½ t mineral or sea salt

Place all ingredients except olive oil into a bottle or jar, close the lid, and shake until well blended. Add olive oil and shake again. Store in refrigerator, and shake well before serving.

Live Caesar Dressing

1 avocado
¼ C ground sunflower seeds
½ -1 clove garlic
3 T lemon juice
Mineral or sea salt to taste
Fresh ground black pepper
Water

Process all ingredients in a blender, adding water as needed to create a creamy dressing.

JUICES, SMOOTHIES, MILKS, AND DRINKS

Note: If sugar imbalances are present, replace carrots and beets in vegetable juices with broccoli, cucumber, or green vegetable of choice, and avoid fruit juices.

Healing Juice

3 carrots
1 beet
3 stalks celery
¼ C fresh parsley
1 bell pepper
¼ inch slice of ginger root
5 kale leaves

Run all ingredients through a juicer, and pour into a tall glass. To increase the healing power of this juice, add a pinch of cayenne powder, or one teaspoon of super-green powder.

Apple Pear Juice

3 medium apples
2 medium pears

Process through juicer, stir well, and serve.

Summer Passion Juice

½ pineapple, peeled and cored
¼ lb fresh cherries, pitted
2 1-inch cubes pineapple
2 whole cherries

Process pineapple and cherries through a juicer. Stir well. Thread pineapple chunks and cherries onto a cocktail skewer. Pour juice into a tall glass, add speared fruit, and enjoy.

Mega-Green Juice

2 stalks celery
1 cucumber
1 zucchini
1 C spinach leaves
1 green bell pepper

Juice all ingredients, stir, and serve.

Super Seven Juice

3 carrots
1 beet
½ cucumber
2 stalks celery
¼ C fresh parsley
½ red bell pepper
5 kale leaves

Juice all ingredients, stir well, and serve.

Mineral Magic Juice

3 carrots
2 stalks celery
¼ C fresh parsley
1 bunch spinach leaves

Juice all ingredients, stir, and serve.

Living Light

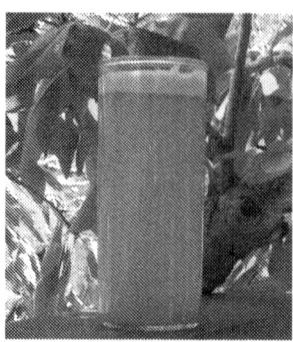

*"Each time we remove a dark thought or feeling,
we are a little closer to greater love, better health,
and to achieving our greater potential."*
Richard Anderson, N.D., N.M.D.[34]

Everyday Detox Juice

3 carrots
2 stalks celery
5-6 dark green leaves
  (spinach, kale, or chard)
¼ C fresh parsley
¼ inch slice of ginger

Juice, stir, and serve.

Powerhouse Smoothie

1 banana
½ mango
6 1-inch pieces of
  fresh pineapple
10 soaked almonds
1 T ground golden flax seed
1 T super-green powder
1 T bee pollen
Water or fruit juice

Place all ingredients in a blender and cover with pure water, or fresh juice. Blend until smooth, and drink immediately.

Banana Coconut Smoothie

1 banana
¼ C grated coconut
Coconut milk
1-inch piece soaked
  vanilla pod
1 T raw honey, optional

Place banana, grated coconut, and vanilla pod in blender. Process slowly, while adding enough coconut milk to create a thick creamy smoothie. Add honey and blend well.

Super Green Smoothie

1 banana
4 figs
1 T super-green powder
1 t chlorella
1 t spirulina
1 T raw honey, optional
Water or apple juice

Blend fruits, powders, and honey with enough water or juice to create a creamy smoothie.

Alkalizing Broth

3 potatoes, chopped
3 stalks celery, chopped
6 kale leaves,
  or 1 C spinach leaves
1 C sea vegetables
1 quart pure water

Bring all ingredients to a boil in a stainless steel pot. Simmer for 20 minutes. Remove from heat and allow the broth to cool. Strain out vegetables, reserving broth. Store in the refrigerator and drink 2 to 3 C daily during preparation week, and on fasting days.

NUT AND SEED MILKS AND CREAMS

To prepare any milk or cream, follow these basic steps:

1. Soak seeds or nuts in pure water for the time indicated in the soaking chart in Chapter Two.

2. Soak any dried fruit that you wish to add for 4-6 hours.

3. Drain nuts, seeds, and soaked fruits. Do not save or drink the soak water from nuts or seeds – it contains toxins. Fruit soak water can be used in recipes.

4. Combine all soaked nuts, seeds, and fruits in a blender along with any flavorings or spices. Add water, coconut milk, or fruit soak water. Use about 2 C nuts/seeds to 1 C liquid. Use less liquid for creams.

5. Process all ingredients in a blender until smooth.

6. Strain the liquid through a fine cheesecloth or nylon mesh over a bowl to catch the milk. You will have to squeeze the pulp to get all the liquid out. You may want to make a straining bag using nylon, cheesecloth, or any small mesh fabric. The bag is easy to wash by hand, and to reuse. Discard the pulp, or save to use in dehydrator bread, cookie, or pie crust recipes.

7. Refrigerating the milk for at least one hour before serving allows all of the flavors to strengthen. However, it can also be used right away. Milk will keep in the refrigerator for 2-3 days.

8. Store in a tightly covered glass jar, and shake well before each use.

Almond Cream

2 C soaked almonds
½ C water
¼ C coconut milk
1 T flax oil
2-inch piece soaked
  vanilla bean
¼ C soaked raisins

Follow instructions above for milks, using only as much water and coconut milk as needed to make the mixture thick and creamy.

Almond Milk

2 C soaked almonds
1 C pure water, coconut
  milk, or coconut water
2-inch length soaked
  vanilla bean
⅛ C soaked raisins

Follow instructions above for milks. This basic recipe can be adjusted to create many tasty drinks. Optional additions include cinnamon, maple syrup, cardamom, ground raw chocolate, carob powder, orange essence, and mint essence. After completion of the Living Light program, try hazelnut milk, pecan milk, cashew milk, and macadamia nut milk.

Sunflower Seed Milk

1 C soaked sunflower seeds
½ C pure water
1-inch length soaked
  vanilla bean
1-2 T soaked raisins to
  sweeten as desired

Blend ingredients together, and strain as detailed in the directions for milks above.

Non-Dairy Kefir

1-2 T Kefir grains
2 C *Nut Milk* or *Seed Milk*
2-3 t orange juice

Place grains in a quart-sized jar. Add orange juice to the *Nut Milk* or *Seed milk* and mix well. Pour the milk into the jar with the grains until it is ¾ full. Cover loosely and let the milk sit at room temperature away from sunlight for 24 hours, or until the milk has coagulated and is sour tasting. Strain through a nylon mesh and reserve the creamy Kefir milk. Kefir milk may be consumed immediately or stored in the refrigerator for a few days to ripen further. Save the residual grains from the mesh strainer in an airtight container, and add to fresh grains as starter for the next batch. Kefir sour cream or yogurt can be made by using less *Nut Milk* or *Seed Milk*.

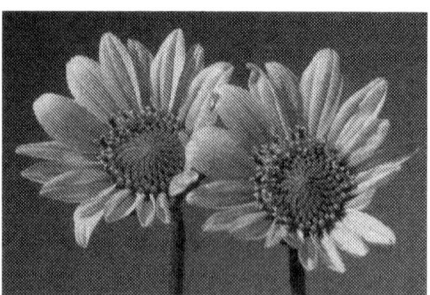

"And you shall feel another spirit awakening within yourself and strengthening you and passing over your entire body and giving you pleasure."
Rabbi Abraham Abulafia[35]

SALADS, SOUPS, AND SIDE DISHES

Basil Bean Salad

1 C sprouted mung beans
1 C sprouted chickpeas
1 C fresh green beans, chopped
½ C sliced black olives
Fresh whole kernel corn sliced from two ears
1 medium red bell pepper, chopped
1 medium shallot, chopped
¼ C apple cider vinegar
¼ C flax oil
2 T chopped fresh basil
1 t chili powder
½ t black pepper
1 t ground mustard powder

In a large bowl, combine sprouts, beans, olives, corn, bell pepper, and shallot. In a small bowl combine vinegar, oil, basil, chili powder, black pepper, and ground mustard, and mix well. Pour vinegar blend over bean mixture, and toss to coat. Chill for several hours or overnight, occasionally stirring or shaking the mixture to marinate. Stir well just before serving.

California Coleslaw

1 C finely sliced green cabbage
¾ C grated carrot
1 green bell pepper, finely diced
1 stalk celery, finely diced
4-5 kale leaves, minced
¼ C *Avonaise*
Mineral or sea salt to taste
Ground black pepper to taste

Mix all vegetables together in a large bowl. Add *Avonaise* and stir thoroughly. Serve immediately, or refrigerate for up to one hour before serving.

Spinach Caesar Salad

1 bunch spinach leaves, washed
½ C sliced black olives
½ C soaked sun-dried tomatoes, diced
Live Caesar Dressing
Pumpkin Parmesan

Chop spinach into bite-sized pieces and place in a large bowl. Add black olives and sun-dried tomatoes. Top with *Live Caesar Dressing* and sprinkle with *Pumpkin Parmesan*.

Greek Salad with Seed Cheese

1 head romaine lettuce, chopped
½ C black olives
1 cucumber, peeled and chopped
1 medium tomato, chopped
1 small green bell pepper, chopped
1 t minced fresh oregano
⅛ C olive oil
Juice of one lemon
Ground black pepper to taste
Seed Cheese

Place lettuce in a large bowl. Combine all remaining ingredients, except *Seed Cheese*, in a medium bowl and mix well. Pour mixed vegetables and seasonings onto lettuce, and toss gently. Top individual servings with a few teaspoon-sized dollops of *Seed Cheese*.

Sprout Salad

1 C alfalfa sprouts
1 C broccoli sprouts
½ C radish sprouts
½ C red clover sprouts
1 C sunflower greens, chopped

Combine all sprouts in a large bowl and mix well. Serve with *Avonaise*.

Garden Salad

2 C chopped lettuce of choice
½ C alfalfa-radish sprout mix
1 tomato, chopped
1 cucumber, peeled and thinly sliced
1 avocado, diced
3 T minced fresh parsley

Place all ingredients in a large bowl and toss lightly. Serve with dressing of choice.

Broccoli and Apple Salad

2 C romaine lettuce or spinach leaves, chopped
½ head broccoli, chopped into bite-sized pieces
2 medium apples, diced
¼ C soaked sunflower seeds
4 T apple cider vinegar

Combine all ingredients except apple cider vinegar in a large bowl. Sprinkle with vinegar, and mix well.

Ocean Salad

1 C mixed field greens
½ C re-hydrated sea vegetable salad mix, rinsed well and chopped
½ C peeled and chopped cucumber
¼ C soaked sesame seeds
Tamari Dressing

Mix all ingredients in a large bowl. Add *Tamari Dressing* and toss well.

Living Light

Cucumber Dill Salad

2 medium cucumbers, peeled and sliced thinly
2 T minced fresh dill
3 T olive oil
Mineral or sea salt to taste
Mixed salad greens

Combine cucumbers, dill, olive oil, and salt in a mixing bowl, and toss well. Place salad greens in a large dish and top with cucumber dill mixture.

Tomato Basil Salad

2-3 medium tomatoes, chopped
¼ C finely chopped fresh basil
3-4 T olive oil
Mineral or sea salt to taste
Fresh salad greens

Toss tomatoes, basil, salt, and olive oil together in a small bowl. Serve over chopped salad greens.

Sesame Kale Salad

6 kale leaves, washed, de-stemmed, and chopped
4 T ground sesame seeds
½ C re-hydrated Arame sea vegetables, rinsed well and chopped
¼ C flax oil
1 T grated ginger
½ clove minced garlic
Mineral or sea salt to taste

Soften kale leaves by rubbing them with salt for a few minutes. Combine kale and sea vegetables in a large bowl. Blend flax oil, sesame seed meal, ginger, garlic and salt in a blender until creamy. Pour sesame-oil over kale and Arame, toss well, and serve.

Creamy Tomato Soup

2 stalks celery, juiced
4 fresh tomatoes
6 soaked sun-dried tomatoes, reserve soak water
¼ C ground sunflower seeds
1 t dried basil
Mineral or sea salt to taste

Place all ingredients in a blender, adding tomato soak water as needed, and process until smooth and creamy.

Cucumber Avocado Soup

1 cucumber
1 avocado
1 C *Rejuvelac*
¼ clove garlic
1 T fresh dill, minced
Mineral or sea salt to taste

Process all ingredients in a blender until well mixed and creamy.

Cilantro Carrot Soup

3 carrots
2 stalks celery
¼ C ground sunflower seeds
¼ C minced fresh cilantro
Mineral or sea salt to taste

Juice carrots and celery. Combine juices in a blender, adding sunflower seed meal to create creamy consistency. Add cilantro and salt, and blend again.

Miso Soup

Mix 1-2 T unpasteurized miso with 1½ C of very warm water (less than 120° F/50° C). Add your choice of grated carrot, minced kale, finely chopped cabbage, chopped sea vegetables, sliced green onions, and diced celery. Stir thoroughly and serve.

Creamy Sweet Potatoes

2 sweet potatoes, peeled and chopped
1 T coconut oil
Mineral or sea salt to taste

Process chopped sweet potatoes through a homogenizing juicer using the solid screen. Blend puréed potatoes with coconut oil and salt in a food processor until smooth and fluffy.

Antipasto Treats

Green, black, and Kalamata olives, pitted
Cherry tomatoes, halved
Sliced green bell peppers
Cauliflower, chopped into bite-sized pieces
Button mushrooms
6 soaked sun-dried tomatoes
½ t each dried basil, oregano, and thyme
½ clove garlic
¼ C olive oil
3 T apple cider vinegar

Place vegetables in a large bowl. Combine sun-dried tomatoes, spices, garlic, olive oil, and vinegar in a blender and process on high until liquefied. Pour antipasto sauce over vegetables, and toss to coat. Marinate covered in the refrigerator overnight, stirring occasionally.

Our Daily Shred

1 carrot
1 beet
¼ head cabbage
1 red bell pepper, diced
2 stalks celery, diced
2 green onions, sliced
2 T minced fresh parsley
Mineral or sea salt to taste

Grate carrot and beet in a food processor, and place in a medium bowl. Thinly slice and chop cabbage, and add to carrot-beet mixture. Add peppers, celery, onions, parsley, and salt. Toss well and serve as a side dish with any meal. *Our Daily Shred* can also be piled onto lettuce leaves or Nori sheets, and folded or rolled to make a tasty lunch or snack.

Recipes

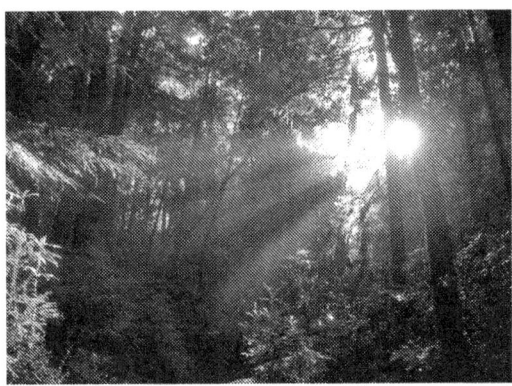

*"He saw the light adhering to his body… and penetrating
all of his limbs…into his entire body, to his heart
and his inward (parts), and (the light)
transformed (him) into fire and light."*
Symeon[36]

Living Light

MAIN DISHES

Almond Seed Pâté

1 C soaked almonds
¼ C soaked pumpkin seeds
¼ C soaked sunflower seeds
1 medium or two small shallots, chopped in quarters
½ clove garlic (optional)
1 stalk celery, minced
1 bell pepper, minced
2 T parsley, chopped
Mineral or sea salt to taste
Fresh ground black pepper
½ T celery seed, rubbed
¼ T thyme
2-4 T flax seed oil

Process nuts, seeds, shallots, and garlic in a homogenizing juicer using the solid plate or screen, or in a food processor with the 'S' blade until smooth. Put nut and seed mixture into a large bowl, and stir in flax oil as needed to create pâté consistency. Add remaining ingredients. Mix well. Cover and refrigerate at least 1 hour before serving. Pâté will keep in the fridge for 2-3 days.

Walnut and Sun-Dried Tomato Pâté

1 C soaked walnuts*
½ C soaked sun-dried tomatoes
½ C finely diced celery
¼ C finely diced shallots
½ C finely diced red bell pepper
1 t celery seeds, rubbed
Sea or mineral salt to taste
Freshly ground black pepper

Process walnuts and sun-dried tomatoes through a homogenizing juicer, using the solid plate or screen. Alternatively, use a food processor with the 'S' blade, and blend to a smooth consistency. Place walnut-tomato mixture in a large bowl. Add all other ingredients and mix well. Refrigerate for at least one hour before serving.
*Replace walnuts with almonds during the Living Light program.

Lunch Tacos

Large cabbage or romaine lettuce leaves
2 tomatoes, chopped
2 carrots, grated
½ avocado, sliced
½ C raw hummus or pâté of choice
Alfalfa sprouts

Spread hummus or pâté on leaves and top with veggies and sprouts. Roll or fold and eat! For variety, add black olives, soaked seeds, or grated beets.

Vegetable Loaf

8 carrots
3 stalks celery, minced
½ C soaked sunflower seeds
1 medium green bell pepper, minced
½ medium onion, minced
2 zucchinis, shredded
½ clove garlic, minced
½ C ground sunflower seeds
¼ C minced fresh parsley
1 t dried basil
Fresh ground black pepper to taste
Mineral or sea salt to taste

Juice carrots, and place the pulp in a large bowl, reserving ¼ C of the juice. Add minced vegetables, seasonings, soaked seeds, and seed meal. Mix well, adding a little juice as needed to make thick moist dough. Form mixture into a loaf shape and dehydrate at 105° F / 40° C for six hours. Slice and serve.

Falafel Balls

2 C chickpea sprouts or soaked almonds
½ onion, minced
½ C fresh parsley, minced
1 clove garlic, minced
1 t cumin
¼ t cayenne pepper
Flax oil

Process all ingredients in a food processor, adding flax oil as needed to form a smooth, thick mixture. Shape into 1-inch balls, and dehydrate at 105° F / 40° C for eight hours. Serve with *Tabouli*, *Raw Hummus*, and *Turkish Flat Bread*.

Spaghetti Squash with Zesty Marinara Sauce

Halve spaghetti squash and remove seeds. Slice into quarters and remove skin. Grate the squash in a food processor. Place grated squash in a dish and cover with water. Let stand for 1 to 2 hours to soften. Drain squash and place in a serving dish. Top with *Zesty Marinara Sauce* and *Pumpkin Parmesan*.

Tabouli

1 C sprouted wheat
¾ C fresh parsley, minced
½ onion, minced
1 medium cucumber, diced
1 medium tomato, chopped
¼ C minced fresh mint
Juice of one lemon
3 T olive oil
3 T apple cider vinegar

Combine all ingredients in a bowl. Cover and refrigerate for at least one hour before serving.

Sunlight Burgers

1 C soaked sunflower seeds
½ C soaked almonds
½ C minced fresh parsley
5 soaked sun-dried tomatoes
½ onion, minced
1 T dried thyme
1 T dried sage
Fresh ground black pepper to taste
Mineral or sea salt to taste
Flax oil

Process soaked seeds, nuts, and sun-dried tomatoes through a homogenizing juicer using the solid plate or screen. Alternatively, process the mixture in a food processor using the 'S' blade. Place seed mix in a large bowl and add remaining ingredients. Stir until well blended, adding flax oil as needed to form into dough that holds together. Shape into patties and dehydrate at 105° F/ 40° C for 8 hours. Serve with salad greens and *Spicy Mexican Salsa*.

Extraordinary Mushroom Pâté

1 C mushrooms, washed and de-stemmed
¼ C soaked sun-dried tomatoes
½ C almonds, soaked
2 stalks celery, minced
1 medium red bell pepper, minced
½ onion, minced
¼ C fresh parsley, minced
2 T fresh basil, minced or 1 T dried basil
Fresh ground black pepper
Mineral or sea salt to taste
Golden flax seed meal

Process mushrooms, almonds, and sun-dried tomatoes through a homogenizing juicer using the solid plate or screen, or purée in a food processor with the 'S' blade. Place mushroom tomato mixture in a bowl and combine with all ingredients except flax seed meal. Stir well, adding flax seed meal 1 tablespoon at a time as needed to create pâté consistency. Store covered in the refrigerator for at least one hour and stir again before serving.

Tossed Chinese Vegetables

1 head broccoli, cut into bite-sized pieces
½ head cauliflower, cut into bite-sized pieces
3 stalks celery, chopped
2 carrots, sliced very thinly
2 C bok choy leaves and stems, sliced thinly
1 medium red bell pepper, chopped
½ C re-hydrated, mixed sea vegetables, chopped finely
1 clove garlic, minced
3 T Tamari sauce
3 T raw Tahini
¼ C chopped fresh cilantro
1 T ginger, minced
4 T ground sesame seeds
4 T flax seed oil

Place vegetables in a large bowl. Combine garlic, Tamari, Tahini, cilantro, ginger, sesame seed meal, and flax seed oil in a small bowl and whisk. Pour sauce over vegetables and stir well. Refrigerate for one hour. Stir well before serving.

Sushi Rolls

Raw Nori sheets (sun-dried, not toasted)
1 C cucumber, sliced into thin 1-inch long strips
1 C carrots, shredded
1 C avocado, thinly sliced
1 C red clover sprouts
1 C *Seed Cheese*

Spread *Seed Cheese* on Nori sheet, covering all but the edges and corners. Place mixed, sliced vegetables across the center. Top with sprouts. Roll Nori from one side into a tight roll. Serve whole or slice into 1-inch thick rounds. Serve with *Tamari Dressing*.

Live Lasagna

4 medium sized zucchinis
1½ C *Seed Cheese*
1 C spinach, minced
1 medium red bell pepper, minced
½ C sliced black olives
1½ C *Zesty Marinara Sauce*
Mineral or sea salt

Slice zucchinis lengthwise into thin strips using a knife or mandolin. Place zucchini strips on a plate and sprinkle with a little mineral or sea salt. Combine spinach, bell pepper, and olives in a medium bowl and mix well. Arrange ingredients in a glass baking dish, alternating layers of zucchini, seed cheese, spinach mix, and marinara sauce. May be served fresh or dehydrated at 125° F/50° C for up to one hour to warm.

Pizza Rounds

1 eggplant, peeled
2 medium tomatoes, sliced thinly
½ C *Seed Cheese*
½ C *Zesty Marinara Sauce*
1 t dried oregano
1 t dried basil
1 t dried rosemary
Mineral or sea salt
Toppings: mushrooms, black olives, chopped bell pepper, chopped onion

Slice eggplant into ¼-inch thick rounds, sprinkle with a little mineral or sea salt, and let stand for one hour. Top each eggplant round with marinara sauce, seed cheese, seasonings, and toppings. Place tomato slice on top. Dehydrate at 105° F / 40° C for 6 to 8 hours, until the pizza rounds are soft and dry.

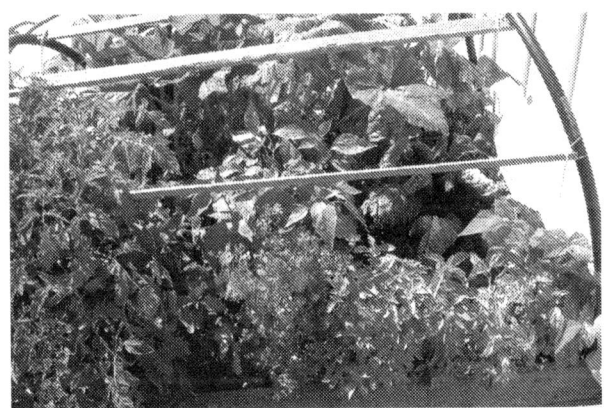

"Let your body seek harmony with the spirit flowing about it, so that the two become one."
The Brotherhood[37]

Living Light

BREAKFAST DISHES

Morning Granola

½ C soaked almonds
½ C soaked pumpkin seeds
½ C soaked sunflower seeds
1 T grade B maple syrup
¼ C shredded coconut
½ C each, chopped apples,
  sliced banana,
  fresh berries
¼ C soaked dried fruit of
  choice, chopped
⅛ t each, cinnamon
  and nutmeg
Flax oil

Process soaked nuts and seeds in a food processor using the 'S' blade, leave the mixture slightly chunky. Place seed and nut mix in a bowl and stir in maple syrup, coconut, and spices. Use a little flax oil to help the mixture stick together slightly. Add fruits and toss lightly. Serve with *Almond Milk* or *Fruigurt*.

Fresh Fruits with Super Seed Mix

1 apple, chopped
1 banana, sliced
1 peach, sliced
½ C red grapes, halved
4 T *Super Seed Mix*

Mix fruits in a bowl and sprinkle with *Super Seed Mix*.

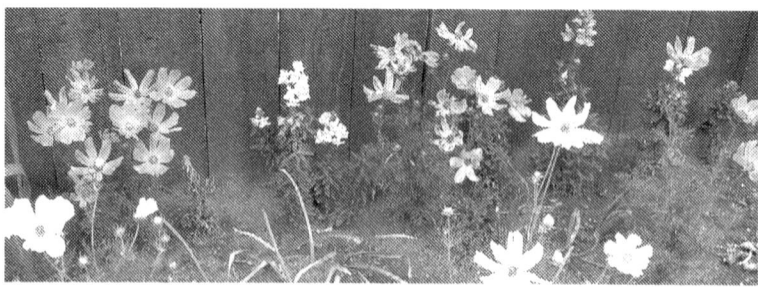

Recipes

Dried Fruit and Seed Granola

½ C soaked sunflower seeds
½ C soaked pumpkin seeds
¼ C ground golden flax seeds
¼ C dried cherries, soaked
¼ C dried blueberries, soaked
¼ C dried cranberries, soaked
¼ t cinnamon
¼ t nutmeg
Mineral or sea salt to taste
Flax seed oil

Process sunflower and pumpkin seeds in a food processor with the 'S' blade, leaving the mixture chunky. Place seed mix in a bowl. Add flax seed meal, dried fruits, and spices, and toss. Add flax seed oil 1 T at a time until the mixture forms into a soft dough-like consistency. Place tablespoons of the mixture on a dehydrator sheet, and dehydrate at 105° F / 40° C for 6 to 8 hours. Stir once or twice so that the granola becomes firm and dry. Store in an airtight container in the refrigerator and serve with *Almond Milk* or *Fruigurt*.

Diced Apples and Raisins

2 apples, diced
½ C soaked raisins
⅛ t pumpkin pie spice
3 T orange juice
4 T *Super Seed Mix*

Place fruits, spice, and orange juice in a bowl and mix well. Sprinkle with *Super Seed Mix*.

Tropical Breakfast

1 C pineapple, chopped
½ C mango, chopped
½ C papaya, chopped
½ C banana, sliced
¼ C coconut, shredded

Place fruits and coconut in a bowl, mix well, and serve.

Wheat Berry Porridge

1 C sprouted wheat
¼ C soaked sunflower seeds
Flax oil or *Almond Milk*
3 T soaked raisins
1 T raw honey, optional
1 T bee pollen

Process wheat and sunflower seeds through a homogenizing juicer using the solid plate or screen, then blend until smooth in a food processor. Add flax oil or *Almond Milk* a few tablespoons at a time and process again to create a creamy porridge consistency. Place wheat porridge in a bowl and stir in raisins, honey, and pollen.

Orange Banana Fruigurt

1 orange
1 banana
3 T ground golden flax seed
3 T flax seed oil
1 T raw honey
Water

Chop fruits and place in blender. Add flax seed oil and honey. Liquefy the mixture until it is thick and creamy, adding water as needed. Fruigurt will continue to thicken after blending. If it is too thick, add more water; if too thin, add more flax seed meal. Serve immediately.

Banana Coconut Fruigurt

1 banana
¼ C coconut, chopped
½ C coconut milk
3 T ground golden flax seed
3 T flax seed oil
2-inch piece soaked
  vanilla bean
1 T raw honey
Water

Place banana and coconut pieces into blender. Add coconut milk, flax seed meal, flax oil, vanilla bean, and honey. Blend until thick and creamy, adding water or flax seed meal as needed to create a yogurt-like consistency. Serve immediately.

Berry Fruigurt

½ C strawberries
½ C blueberries
¼ C raspberries
3-4 T ground golden
   flax seed
3 T flax seed oil
1 T raw honey
Water

Blend berries, flax seed meal, flax seed oil, and honey in blender. Adjust water and flax seed meal to create a thick and creamy texture. Serve immediately.

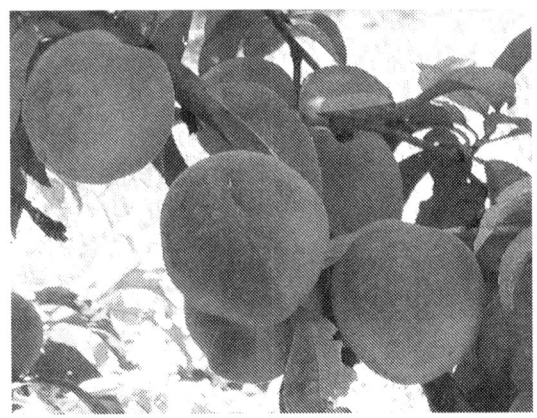

*"Our everyday life needs to be transformed
into a spiritual sanctuary."*
Gabriel Cousens, M.D.[38]

CRACKERS, CHIPS, AND BREADS

Note: Store dehydrated foods in airtight containers in the refrigerator. They will keep for up to one month.

Corn Chips

4 ears of fresh corn
½ small onion, minced
¾ C soaked sunflower seeds
Mineral or sea salt to taste
Water

Slice corn from cob and place in a blender with the other ingredients. Blend until smooth, adding a little water as needed to make a thick batter. Place tablespoons of batter on dehydrator sheets, shaping into rounds or triangles. Dehydrate at 105° F / 40° C for 12 to 16 hours or until the chips are dry and crisp.

Flax Crackers

2 C golden flax seeds
1 medium red bell pepper, minced
½ t oregano
½ t thyme
½ t basil
Mineral or sea salt to taste
Water

Soak flax seeds in pure water for 5 hours or until the mixture becomes gelatinous. Place soaked seeds in a mixing bowl and stir in minced pepper and seasonings. Spread the mixture thinly onto dehydrator sheets, wetting hands or spatula as needed to keep it from sticking. Dehydrate at 105° F / 40° C for 6 hours, then turn the mixture over and remove the dehydrator sheets. Continue dehydrating for an additional 5 to 6 hours until dry and crisp. Break into serving size crackers. A variety of seasonings can be added to the basic recipe including chili powder, garlic, and dill.

Essene Bread

2 C sprouted wheat or rye
¼ C ground golden
 flax seeds

Process soaked grain through a homogenizing juicer using the solid plate or screen, or purée in a food processor into a thick dough. Shape dough into a thick round or loaf shape, and coat with flax seed meal to reduce surface stickiness. Dehydrate at 105° F/ 40° C for 12 to 16 hours until the loaf is dry on the outside and soft and warm on the inside. Alternatively, place the loaf into the bowl of a slow-cooker and heat on low for 10 hours.

Nori Crackers

Raw Nori sheets
1 C *Seed Cheese*
1 avocado, mashed
Mineral or sea salt to taste

Cut Nori sheets into 3-inch x 3-inch squares. Combine seed cheese, avocado, and salt in a bowl and mix well. Spread cheese and avocado mixture onto Nori squares. Dehydrate at 105° F/ 40° C for 6 hours or until crackers are dry.

Turkish Flat Bread

1 C sprouted rye
1 C sprouted lentils
¼ t caraway seeds
½ onion, minced
¼ C Tahini
Mineral or sea salt to taste
Water

Process rye and lentils through a homogenizing juicer with solid plate or screen, or grind in a food processor until dough forms, adding a little water as needed. Place dough into a mixing bowl and add caraway, onion, Tahini, and salt. Mix thoroughly, adding water as needed while maintaining thickness. Form dough into thin 5-inch rounds and place on dehydrator sheets. Dehydrate at 105° F/ 40° C for 6 hours then flip rounds, and continue dehydrating for 5 to 6 hours until dry.

Garlic Seed Bread

1 C soaked pumpkin seeds
1 C *Seed Cheese*
1 clove garlic, minced
¼ C fresh parsley, minced
½ onion, minced
Flax seed meal
Mineral or sea salt to taste

Process pumpkin seeds through a homogenizing juicer using the solid plate or screen, or purée in a food processor until creamy. Place mashed seeds in a bowl and mix with seed cheese, garlic, parsley, onion, and salt. Add flax meal as needed to form soft dough. Shape dough into ¼-inch thick 2-inch by 4-inch rectangles. Place on dehydrator trays and dehydrate at 105° F/ 40° C for 6 to 8 hours until dry and soft.

FERMENTED FOODS

Sauerkraut

1 head cabbage
1 clove garlic, minced
1 t dried dill
1 t mineral or sea salt

Remove and save outer leaves of the cabbage. Juice half of the cabbage; finely slice and chop the other half. Mix juice, pulp, shredded cabbage, garlic, dill, and salt together, and place in a large glass or ceramic bowl. Cover with the outer leaves of the cabbage. Place a large plate on top of the mixture, and set a heavy weight on top. Leave at room temperature for 3 or 4 days until it tastes tangy and sour. In warm weather, fermentation may only take two days. Store in a covered container in the refrigerator.

Beet Relish

3 beets
1 stalk celery, diced
½ C sauerkraut
¼ inch slice ginger root, grated
¼ C fresh cilantro, minced

Juice two beets, and finely grate the third one. Combine beet juice, pulp, and shredded beet in a bowl with remaining ingredients and mix well. Store in refrigerator for several hours before serving.

Crispy Pickles

2 large cucumbers
½ onion, sliced thin
1 T dill seed, rubbed
1 T dill leaves
1 small green bell pepper, minced
1 t mineral or sea salt
1 C sauerkraut

Peel cucumbers and slice into thin rounds. Place in a large, wide-mouthed jar, and add pepper, onions, dill seeds and leaves, and salt. Process sauerkraut in a blender or food processor until well minced. Strain through cheesecloth or mesh, reserving juice. Discard sauerkraut pulp, or return to the sauerkraut mix. Pour sauerkraut juice into the jar with cucumbers, cover, and shake. Refrigerate overnight.

Rejuvelac

1 C sprouted wheat or rye
3 C pure water

Blend grain with water, and pour into a large jar. Cover with mesh or sprouting screen. Leave at room temperature for 2 to 3 days until the taste is tart. Strain mixture, reserving the liquid, and refrigerate in a covered jar. May be used in recipes or enjoyed as a refreshing healthy drink. Alternative sprouted grains may be used including millet, rice, barley, or buckwheat.

Recipes

SEED CHEESE AND TOPPINGS

•⋯⋯⋯⋯Seed Cheese⋯⋯⋯⋯•

1 C sunflower seeds, soaked overnight
½ C sesame seeds
2 C water

Drain and rinse sunflower seeds. Grind sesame seeds into a fine powder. Place sunflower seeds and sesame seed meal in a blender. Add water while blending to a creamy consistency. Pour into a glass container or bowl, and cover with a cloth. Let stand at room temperature for 8 to 12 hours, or until the mixture separates into solid "cheese" and watery "whey", and bubbles form on top. It will have a sour lemony taste. Strain through a cheesecloth bag and discard the liquid. Hang the bag of cheese over a bowl in the refrigerator overnight. Remove the dry seed cheese from the bag, and store in an airtight container in the refrigerator. Cheese may be thinned into a cheese sauce by adding water to create the desired consistency.

•⋯⋯⋯⋯Super Seed Mix⋯⋯⋯⋯•

½ C sunflower seeds
½ C pumpkin seeds
½ C golden flax seeds

Grind seeds in a coffee/spice grinder into a fine meal. Place the seed meal in an airtight container, mix well, and seal. Store in the refrigerator and serve on fruits, salads, vegetables, and soups.

Living Light

Pumpkin Parmesan

Grind ¼ C pumpkin seeds in a coffee/spice grinder. Sprinkle liberally on salads, raw pasta and pizza dishes, and fresh fruit.

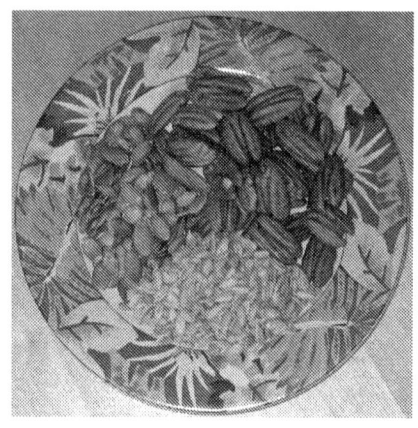

*"To change your mood or mental state,
change your vibration"*
The Kybalion[39]

DESSERTS AND TREATS

Note: These foods are great for special events, holidays, and as occasional treats. It is advisable to avoid them during the Living Light program, and to limit sweet snacks in the diet to once or twice a week after the program.

Moon Balls

2 C dates
2 C soaked pecans
½ C raisins
1 t cinnamon
1 t grated lemon peel
1 T orange juice
Shredded raw coconut
Finely chopped
    soaked pecans

Process dates, pecans, and raisins through a homogenizing juicer using the solid plate or screen. Place in a bowl, add cinnamon, lemon peel, and orange juice, and mix well. Form the mixture into 1-inch balls, and roll through mixed coconut and chopped pecans. For variety, try adding raw chocolate or carob powder in place of cinnamon for chocolate flavored *Moon Balls*, or add a 2-inch length of soaked vanilla bean and 1 T maple syrup for a rich delight.

Chocolate Fudge

1 C dates
½ C ground raw chocolate
    or raw chocolate
    powder
2 T coconut oil
½ C soaked walnuts,
    chopped
Ground flax seed
    as needed

Process dates and ¼ C of the walnuts through a juicer, using the solid plate or screen. Place date mash in a large bowl. Add coconut oil, chocolate powder, and remaining chopped walnuts, and mix thoroughly. If the mixture is too sticky, add a little ground flax seed meal. Shape mixture into 1-inch squares, place on a platter or plate, cover and refrigerate.

Apple Nutmeg Delight

4 apples, chopped
½ C soaked hazel nuts, pecans, or walnuts, chopped
½ t nutmeg
¼ C *Almond Cream*

Place apples, nuts, and nutmeg in a large bowl. Pour *Almond Cream* over all, and mix well. This dish may be eaten during the Living Light program when made with almonds rather than other nuts.

Cherry Vanilla Trail Mix Bars

1 C soaked almonds
½ C soaked pumpkin seeds
½ C soaked dried cherries, or fresh chopped, pitted cherries
4 dates
¼ C shredded fresh coconut
2-inch piece soaked vanilla bean
Golden flax seed meal

Process almonds, half the pumpkin seeds, dates, and vanilla bean in a homogenizing juicer using the solid plate or screen. Place almond seed mixture in a bowl and add remaining ingredients, using enough flax seed meal to form soft dough. Shape into ¼-inch thick rectangular bars and dehydrate 8 to 10 hours at 105° F/ 40° C until dry and firm. Store the trail bars in an airtight container in the refrigerator.

Chocolate Covered Strawberries

Fresh whole strawberries
½ C finely ground
  raw chocolate
Very warm water
  (not over 120° F/50° C)
2-3 dates
Olive oil

Wash strawberries and pat dry. Cream dates through homogenizing juicer. Mix ground chocolate with dates, and blend with very warm water into a thick sauce. Dip strawberries into chocolate sauce, coating them almost to the stem. Place on a plate coated with olive oil to prevent sticking, or on waxed paper. Refrigerate until chocolate becomes firm.

Chocolate Chip Cookies

1 C almond pulp from
  Almond Milk preparation
¼ C raw chocolate nibs,
  chopped finely
¼ C soaked raisins,
  reserve soak water
2-inch piece soaked
  vanilla bean

Process soaked raisins and vanilla bean through a homogenizing juicer using the solid plate or screen. Place raisin vanilla mixture and almond pulp in a bowl, and stir well to form dough. Mix in chocolate nibs. Add a little raisin soak water if needed to moisten the dough. Form into 2-inch round cookies, and place on dehydrator sheets. Dehydrate at 105° F/ 40° C for 6 hours or until dry and soft.

Mixed Berry Pie

Crust:
2 C soaked pecans
½ C soaked raisins

Process nuts and raisins in a homogenizing juicer using the solid plate or screen. Turn into bowl and mix well. Press into 9-inch pie plate. Refrigerate.

Filling:
½ C sliced strawberries
½ C blueberries
½ C raspberries
½ C blackberries
4 T raw honey
Ground golden flax seeds

Set aside some of each berry for the topping. Process the remaining berries in a blender or food processor with the honey and enough flax seed meal to thicken. Pour berry mix into the crust and arrange leftover berries on top. Refrigerate for several hours before serving. Serve topped with tablespoons of thick *Almond Cream*.

Banana Sundae

2 bananas, peeled and chopped into thirds
¼ C ground raw chocolate or raw chocolate powder
Very warm water (not over 120° F)
4 T soaked nuts of choice, chopped
4 T grated coconut
2 cherries with stems

Freeze banana pieces in an airtight bag or container. Mix raw chocolate powder with a little warm water to form a thick sauce. Process frozen bananas through a homogenizing juicer using the solid plate or screen, catching the "ice cream" in serving dishes. Pour chocolate sauce over ice cream. Top with chopped nuts, grated coconut, and cherries.

Date and Walnut Cake

1 C soaked walnuts
½ C soaked dates
Extra soaked dates and walnuts, chopped

Process nuts and dates through a homogenizing juicer with the solid plate or screen. Mix well. Add extra chopped walnuts and dates, and mix again. Form into small cakes and refrigerate in a covered container for several hours. Serve topped with thick *Almond Cream*.

Chapter Five

Alchemical Yoga
Living Light Meditations

THE MAGIC OF ALCHEMY

"I will show you the power of the Sacred Light."
The Book of Purifying Fire[40]

Alchemy is an ancient philosophy of transformation that is in many ways the Western equivalent of the yoga traditions of the East.[41] Both of these disciplines deal with Vital Essence in its cosmic and personal forms. On the personal level Vital Essence is responsible for the health of the physical body. When all Vital Essence leaves the body the result is death. When it is reduced or constricted, disease and illnesses set in. Consequently, in the beginning stages of Alchemy the focus is on clearing obstructions from the body and healing physical disorders.

Alchemy can be defined as *magical power applied to the process of transmutation*. The magical power that is used in Alchemy is Vital Essence. To transmute is to change something from one state or condition into another. As a part of directing Vital Essence to cleanse the body, its presence must be cultivated and increased. A diet of 100% living foods enables more Vital Essence to accumulate in the body, which fuels the process of physical purification. In addition, specific alchemical meditations and yoga practices accelerate this healing process, and speed reconstruction of the cells and organs of the body.

In the ancient traditions, Alchemy was taught as a sacred discipline that was designed to take one as far beyond the realm of physical change as one desired. Advanced alchemical practices are designed to encourage a state of *illumination*. As an outcome of alchemical practice, illumination means to *be* the light referred to in the quote from *The Book of Purifying Fire* above. The powers of this sacred light include the enhanced awareness, self-mastery, and keen perceptions that may be awakened by the conscious use of alchemical light.

In the techniques of *Alchemical Yoga*, transmutation is accomplished by directly accessing spiritual light with the mind and imagination, and imbedding it deeply into the cells of the body. In the *Alchemical Yoga* meditations presented here, the light is used to create changes to the molecular and atomic structure of the physical being. Because the physical body anchors the emotional, mental, and etheric bodies, any changes that occur therein initiate a chain of cause and effect, radiating greater harmony into every level of being.

Like yoga, alchemical practices focus on opening and balancing the seven primary centers of force in the etheric body[42]. These centers, known as the chakras in the East, are termed the seven interior *stars* or *lamps* by the alchemists. This terminology again points to the universal light as the essential substance in alchemical work. The interior stars were named after the seven planets of the ancients, and likened to seven metals with which the alchemists worked. These associations to the Eastern chakra system are shown in the table below. In the process of alchemical self-transformation, the energy emanating from within the interior stars becomes more consistent and refined.

Over time the improved alignment and finer rate of vibration in the interior stars will establish physical and emotional well being, and may ultimately lead to the activation of a deep intuition that can serve as a source of preeminent knowledge and wisdom. This personal upward shift in the rate of vibration naturally impacts those nearby in a positive and healing way. The first result that occurs as the interior stars awaken; however, is the healing and stabilization of the physical, mental, and emotional aspects of one's own being. The goal of alchemical practice is *equilibration*, a precise balancing of the mind, emotions, and body that leads to greater health and consciousness, and a happier outlook on life.

In yoga the sacred light of Alchemy is called *Kundalini*, a Sanskrit word meaning *coiled up* or *coiling like a snake*. Alchemists likewise have called this force the *serpent power*. This symbolic language refers to the reservoir of Vital Essence that lies coiled at the base of the spine, and remains dormant in most people. In both yoga and Alchemy the sleeping serpent is awakened and raised step-by-step through the interior stars. This force moves upward as an undulating vibration, much like the slithering movement of a snake.

The serpent power can be stimulated by being in the presence of an alchemical *adept*. An adept is one who has completed the *Great Work* of personal transformation, and is known as a *yogi* (male) or *yogini* (female) in the East. Activation of this force may also be accomplished alone using alchemical methods to open and clear the body, and engage the powers of the mind and imagination to arouse and elevate the serpent power.

The Seven Interior Stars

Chakra	**Location**	**Planet**	**Metal**
Root	Base of the spine	Saturn	Lead
Sacral	Sacrum	Mars	Iron
Solar Plexus	Diaphragm	Jupiter	Tin
Heart	Sternum	Sun	Gold
Throat	Base of the skull	Venus	Brass
Third Eye	Forehead/Pineal Gland	Moon	Silver
Crown	Top of the Head	Mercury	Mercury

The light of Alchemy is also referred to as the *essence of fire*, which highlights the ability of Vital Essence to burn away all that is not divine. This fiery force is engaged and supported in the physical body by the consumption of high-energy raw foods that stimulate the digestion and assimilation of greater nutrition, and the elimination of unwanted residues and toxins. This diet is one of the most important keys to equilibrating the body and perfecting the balance of the three natural phases seen throughout worldly life: creation, destruction, and renewal.

Certain *Alchemical Yoga* meditations make use of mental images of fiery light in order to access a vibratory heat that can incinerate conditioned beliefs, erroneous messages, and emotional attachments, and initiate a deep process of holistic regeneration. By applying the principles and methods of Alchemy, the underlying patterns upon which the physical form is built may be improved, allowing the positive changes that are introduced into the body by diet to be sustained, and creating a new foundation for future enhancements and regeneration.

Some of the techniques of *Alchemical Yoga* have been organized into specialized meditations and yoga practices for use during the Living Light program. They are primarily designed to purify the body and renew the mind. Yet they also serve as foundational practices for later techniques that transmute the personality and body into a true living temple. At any level of use, however, the goal of these disciplines is always the improvement and renewal of body, mind, and soul. Regular practice leads to wholeness, the true meaning of healing, wherein all aspects of being are energized and restored.

The *Alchemical Yoga* practices designed for the Living Light program require no specialized knowledge of meditation, yoga, or Alchemy. They are safe to use on one's own, and will slowly and steadily increase physical energy and mental sharpness, and contribute to an overall feeling of peace and joy. The practices include visual meditations, breathing exercises, and gentle yoga movements and stretches that encourage flexibility and strength.

Living Light Meditations

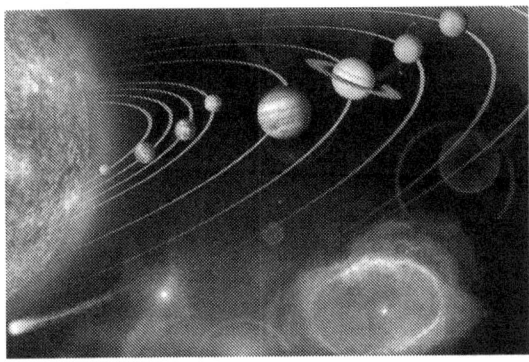

"For the wise man must be as a precious stone; a center of light to all that approach him; giving joy to others because he contains the image of the highest joy in himself; desiring nothing of the world, drawing his inspiration from the supernal light..."
Florence Farr[43]

MEDITATING WITH THE LIVING LIGHT

The *Alchemical Yoga* meditations used during the Living Light Program draw upon traditional alchemical principles to stimulate healing and regeneration. Meditation is the practice of turning the mind and senses away from the outer world, and focusing the attention inward toward the subtle flow of conscious cosmic energy. *Alchemical Yoga* meditations concentrate the mind on detailed configurations of moving light to help turn it from the outer senses, while at the same time creating new and constructive outlets for one's mental energy. These meditations can work miracles when used consistently. They offer a way to harness powerful spiritual energy and direct it toward the transformation of the human body, mind, and emotions.

The central component in all alchemical meditations is the sacred light. The light is envisioned in several specific patterns and colors, each designed for a particular purpose. The meditations rely upon the power of imagination, and the ability to create and sustain visualization. In Alchemy, imagination is defined as *the power of forming images in the mind*, which requires the development of concentration. As the Living Light meditations are mastered, the skills of mental concentration and imagination become sharper as the attention is focused on interesting and beneficial visual imagery.

Concentration can be thought of as the application of one's will to maintain a definite mental focus. While willful intention is a preliminary step in disciplined meditation, the concept of concentration also implies the accumulation, intensification, and consolidation of great energetic force. This energy is fixed, held, and directed by the presence of defined *thought-forms*.

Thought-forms are creations made by both the universal and individual, human minds. They are generated whenever a thought is held in mind unwaveringly. They are strengthened by emotional energy, and on the human level, thought-forms typically come into being without any conscious intent or awareness of their existence. A thought-form is a non-physical yet tangible configuration of mental energy. Examples of universal thought-forms include angels, demons, dragons, fairies, spirits, gods, and goddesses. The strength and clarity of the thought determines the power and duration of the form.

Though they are invisible, consciously created thought-forms can endure for centuries, and their effects upon physical matter are tremendous. One has only to recall the many stories of humans who have experienced assistance from angels to see the power of deliberate thought-forms influencing the reality of material life. In addition to universal thought-forms such as angels, each individual also creates, consciously or unconsciously, a variety of personal mental constructions that impact one's daily life for good or for bad. Personal thought-forms typically manifest in health challenges, the surrounding environment and circumstances of daily life, and unconscious patterns that are repeated in interpersonal relationships.

The concept of thought-forms in Alchemy derives from the Hermetic philosophy of ancient Egypt and Greece. This philosophy is named for the legendary master and teacher Hermes Trismegistus, whose many writings formed the foundation for the Alchemy of the Middle Ages. Hermetic philosophy is also considered to have influenced every religion in existence, yet it transcends all religion as well.

The first principle of Hermetic philosophy is: *All is Mind, the Universe is Mental*, and it further holds that *the phenomenal world or universe is… a mental creation of the All*. The important idea to grasp from this principle is that the human being is a microcosm of the *universal, infinite, living mind*, and can apply the laws of mental creation within his/her own life to create more desirable circumstances. Whatever is created by the power of the mind will ultimately manifest on the physical plane.[44]

The ability to create positive and beneficial thought-forms that lead to health and happiness is aided by developing the skills of mental concentration and imagination, which occurs as one works with alchemical meditations as part of a daily discipline. Daily discipline is easily established when it reflects one's true priorities. Self-improvement, a healthier, slimmer body, greater physical and mental energy, and enhanced spiritual connections are among the many rewards to be gained through the regular practice of concentrating on alchemical imagery.

Concentration is focusing the mind on one thing to the exclusion of everything else. The mind becomes one-pointed, remaining fully absorbed completely with the subject or object of attention. Such single-minded awareness concentrates the Vital Essence into one's intention in a powerful way. Just as a magnifying glass turns the sun's rays into fire when it is properly aligned and focused, so the mind ignites its creative powers through the process of concentration.

The habit-mind is constantly generating thoughts and ideas, most of which are aimless or unfocused, and which contribute to states of stress, worry, and unease. On its simplest level, concentration on alchemical imagery helps relieve the endless stream of mental chatter by diverting mental energy into a specific focus. The act of meditative concentration has been proven to alleviate the effects of physical, mental, and emotional stress and soothe the mind.

In alchemical meditation, a subtler, deeper

mechanism is also at work, capturing and reforming this abundant mental energy into visual forms that serve as seeds from which future improvements on the physical plane will spring. The ability to concentrate also strengthens the will, increases self-confidence, and enhances the benefits of meditation. The exercises below will help improve concentration.

Practices for Developing Concentration

Set a goal to devote 10 minutes each day to concentration practice. Work with each exercise for three or four days before going on to the next one. Begin by sitting on the floor or in a chair with your spine straight. Take three deep breaths and relax.

Exercise 1

Close your eyes and silently repeat the word "peace" in your mind for 5 minutes to start, and work up to 10 minutes. If other thoughts enter your mind, gently but firmly return to repeating "peace".

Exercise 2

Choose any object such as an apple, flower, or seashell. Look at the object steadily and concentrate all of your attention on observing it. Resist all thoughts, even thoughts about the object. Continue to visually examine the object for 5 minutes.

Visualize the same apple or object in your mind. Keep the object nearby and start by looking at it. Then close your eyes and create the object in detail as an inner image. Open your eyes and look at the object if needed. Then close your eyes and visualize it again. Hold the inner image of the object for 5 minutes.

Exercise 3

Draw a circle and color it blue. Look at this image steadily without thought. Let the image be your only focus for a few minutes. Close your eyes and visualize the blue circle. Concentrate only on the blue circle without thinking. If your mind wanders, gently return your attention to the blue circle, and hold this image for the remainder of the 10 minute practice.

Exercise 4

Close your eyes and spend 10 minutes in complete mental silence with no thoughts and no images. If you become aware of thoughts, simply return to silence. This practice may take several attempts to accomplish. Stay with it, and it will become easier each time.

Alchemical Yoga meditations also rely upon and develop the imaginative abilities, which in the science of Alchemy are considered to play a critical role in the human's ability to change existing conditions and create new circumstances in life. In children the imagination is fully free; however, over time most children are encouraged by adults to set aside the joyful experience of imagining as it is commonly dismissed as frivolous, unreal, and deceptive. Consequently, many adults have lost touch with the imaginative powers of the mind. This inherent creative capacity may be reawakened and directed to the attainment of one's desired goals by the prescribed visualizations of Alchemy.

Imagination involves the cultivation and strengthening of an idea that begins as a passive thought. This core idea becomes creative imagination when it is intensified by desire and will. Desire activates the serpent power, and the will directs this force toward the manifestation of the idea on the physical plane. Though the creative aspect of this process operates subconsciously, it requires the conscious intention and focus that attend the regular practice of visual meditations such as those used in *Alchemical Yoga*.

In the beginning of meditation practice it may seem that one is not actually seeing the images in the mind. This is often due to a lack of consciously perceiving the images that are in fact being formed by mentally focusing on the chosen idea. Do not discourage your efforts with negative thoughts such as "I cannot visualize". Visualization is natural and occurs for everyone during dreams. It is only a matter of deliberately making the images conscious. This is best accomplished by adding sensory input into the images. For example, if one imagines sunlight, the experience should include the tactile feeling of warmth and the scent of fresh air in addition to the vision of bright light.

A Simple Technique for Improving Visualization

1. Choose any natural object such as a fruit, flower, stone, or seashell and place it in front of you.
2. Sit in a comfortable position and look carefully at the object.
3. Describe the object out loud and in detail, including shape, colors, texture, smell, etc.
4. Repeat the description a few times.
5. Close your eyes and again describe the object out loud while attempting to see it in your mind's eye. Recreate the object mentally as clearly as possible.
6. Repeat the description and inner visualization of the object for five to ten minutes.
7. Stop the exercise if you become frustrated or bored, and try it again later.

If you feel that you cannot perceive the images described for meditation, it is important to keep in mind that the practices will still be effective. It is the focused intention of the mind and the activation of desire that are most important to success. It is possible to work through the visualizations mentally, and to pretend that the images are being seen. Have faith that the practices will bring positive results, and it will be so.

To the greatest degree possible, imagine the meditative creations in three dimensions and visualize the activity as taking place within and around your body. At first it may only be possible to perceive the imagery in front of your field of vision, and it may look like you are watching yourself as a separate object upon which the actions are taking place. Persevere with the visualizations, working each time to bring the imagery into your body and endeavoring to physically feel the impact and movements of the energy.

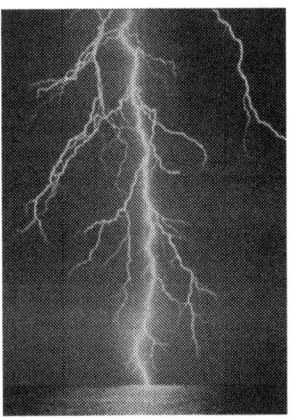

"Imagination is the door leading out of any given situation into another."
Paul Foster Case[45]

The skills of mental concentration and imagination become stronger as one's attention is absorbed with the positive and beneficial thought-forms used in the Living Light meditations. As the visualizations are memorized and mastered, tangible effects begin to appear. The body becomes healthier as it steadily discards its previous toxic form, while the mind and emotions radiate greater peace and optimism. The will power is strengthened, allowing one to manifest success in every aspect of life.

Choose a quiet place for your daily meditation practices, and always meditate in this location. This can be as simple as sitting in the same chair each day. Whenever possible it is also helpful to create a meditation altar with a candle, some incense, flowers, and a spiritually inspiring image. Meditating in the same place each day allows the

Living Light

energy to build up and makes each practice session more productive. It also conditions the mind to enter the meditative state more quickly.

Begin each meditation session with the *Four Count Breath* and *Relaxation Exercise* as outlined below. The *Four Count Breath* attunes the mind to the Kabbalistic cycle of creation, and aligns the body to the four elements of nature: fire, water, air, and earth. Conscious relaxation of the muscles encourages the release of stress and tension, enhances concentration, and enables greater clarity in visualizations. The *Four Count Breath* and *Relaxation Exercise* can also be practiced at any time throughout the day to increase cellular oxygenation and restore balance to the body and mind.

Four Count Breath

Inhale to a slow count of four. Hold the breath in for a slow count of four. Exhale to a slow count of four. Hold the breath out for a slow count of four. Repeat four times.

RELAXATION EXERCISE

Get into a comfortable sitting position with the spine straight. Do not lie down unless you are performing the exercise as a prelude to sleep. Close your eyes, and visualize a pitcher containing crystalline blue liquid just above your head. See the vessel tip over and the liquid begin to flow into the top of your head. This vibrant blue substance brings deep relaxation into everything it touches. See and feel the fluid entering into your head and face, and feel all of the muscles relax as it flows into each area of the body.

As the fluid continues to flow down through the body, all tension is released from the muscles. Continue watching and feeling the relaxing blue liquid moving down through the body, and mentally acknowledge each part of the body as it relaxes, i.e., "my neck is relaxed, my shoulders are relaxed, my arms are relaxed, etc." Finally, see and feel the blue fluid flow out through the bottoms of the feet and relax the feet and toes.

Next, formulate the image of a small black dot in the mind's eye. Imagine writing your first name with this dot. Then write the word, *Relax*. Write your last name with the dot, and then again write the word, *Relax*. Dismiss the image of the dot. Drift quietly and peacefully into silence for a few moments before beginning meditation.

The first meditation in the Living Light program is the *Purifying Light* meditation. This meditation is performed daily during preparation week, and also serves as the foundational practice for all of the visualizations that follow. You should be able to perform the *Purifying Light* meditation with ease before proceeding with the other meditations described below. You may wish to use the *Living Light Alchemical Meditations* CD, which will guide you through all of the practices and visualizations of the Living Light program. See the Appendix for ordering information.

The meditations are undertaken in a progressive manner so that each practice session builds upon the accomplishments of the previous work. A specific meditation designed to enhance the process of cleansing and regenerating the body is performed during each week of the program. A special meditation is used on fasting day each week. Some of the meditations are also used as a component of the *Alchemical Yoga* exercises described in Chapter Six.

The meditations are done daily, and will initially take 30 to 45 minutes to complete, with less time being needed once the imagery is memorized. The visualizations will become easier and more effective each day they are practiced. The meditations are ideally done upon arising in the morning before yoga, exercise, and the *Morning Elixir* drink. They may be repeated at midday, and again in the evening if desired. Once a day is sufficient to attain results; however, the more one practices the meditations, the greater the effects.

PREPARATION WEEK MEDITATION
Purifying Light

Sit in a comfortable position in a chair or on the floor with your spine straight. Close your eyes and inhale deeply, all the way to the bottom of your spine. Slowly exhale, contracting the abdomen, and feel the breath slowly move up and out of the body. Repeat this deep breath twice more.

See in your mind's eye, a sphere nine inches in diameter, made of brilliant, bright, white light sitting at the top of your head. As you visualize this sphere, see it become more radiant. Imagine the white light as *living* light, see it sparkle and crackle with vibrant energy. Focus on increasing the intensity and action of the sphere of white light for a few minutes.

When you are ready, visualize a stream of white light emanating from the sphere. Imagine this stream of living light flowing onto and into the top of your head, as if the sphere had poured liquid light over you. See the liquid light flowing into your head, and immersing your skull and face in brilliant white light. Work carefully with the imagery until you can see the flesh, bones, brain, eyes, ears, etc., pulsating with vivid white light.

Visualize the stream of light continuing to pour down into your body: into your neck and shoulders, down your arms, hands, and fingers, into your chest, upper back, abdomen, pelvis, and hips, through your legs, and out of the bottoms of your feet. Take your time with the image of the flow, and let your attention dwell on each area as it is saturated with brilliant white light. As the light flows out through your feet, consciously direct it to take away all impurities, toxins, and negativity.

See all of your vital organs completely bathed in liquid light. Imagine the white light permeating every cell and molecule of your body. Hold this image in mind, and increase its intensity until you begin to feel your body vibrating in the light.

Meditate on being physically absorbed into the light for several minutes, knowing that the light will rejuvenate and regenerate your body, mind, and soul.

When you feel ready, release all visualizations, and meditate quietly without deliberately generating any thoughts or images. Simply be aware of the feelings in your body and on the surface of your skin where it contacts the air around you. Breathe deeply again three times, becoming conscious of yourself in the room where you are seated. Slowly open your eyes.

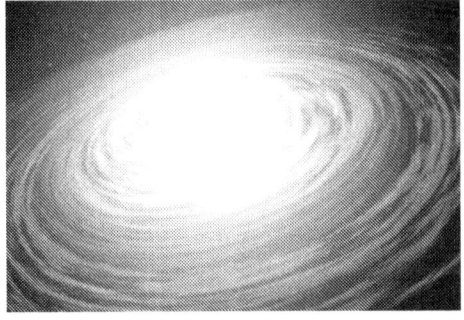

"If you become light, the light will share with you."
The Gospel of Philip[46]

WEEK ONE MEDITATION

Lighting the Seven Lamps

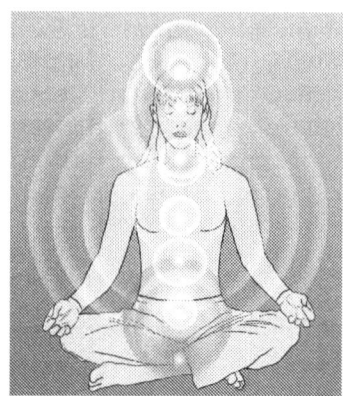

1. Perform the *Four Count Breath* and *Relaxation Exercise*.
2. Perform the *Purifying Light* meditation.
3. Close your eyes. Focus your awareness on the Saturn center at the base of the spine. Visualize a nine-inch sphere of radiant red light centered at the perineum.[47] Continue to meditate on this brilliant red ball of living light, and see it swirling and vibrating with energy. Meditate on the Saturn center for several minutes.
4. Bring your awareness to the Mars center, halfway between the naval and the pubic bone. Visualize this center as a radiant nine-inch sphere of violet light. Meditate on this vibrant violet sphere, seeing it pulsate and glow with living energy. Continue to visualize the Mars center for some time.
5. Move your consciousness to your solar plexus and visualize the Jupiter center as a nine-inch sphere of emerald green light emanating outward in every direction. See this dazzling emerald globe vibrate and expand with dynamic force. Meditate for a while on the green sphere of Jupiter.
6. Bring the focus to your heart and imagine the Sun center as a sphere of intense golden-yellow light, radiating

Living Light Meditations

in all directions. See and feel this glorious gold light as a living force of energy. Focus on this image of the yellow sphere in your heart for several minutes.

7. At the throat, create an image of a bright blue sphere of light. Focus your whole attention on the Venus center as it is bathed in the vital energy of the blue sphere. Meditate steadily on the blue sphere of Venus.

8. Focus your awareness on the Moon center between the eyebrows and centered in the middle of the head. See this center as a nine-inch sphere of luminous indigo light. Visualize this indigo sphere as powerful energetic light, and watch as it glimmers and glows in all directions. Hold the image of the indigo sphere for several minutes.

9. Allow your consciousness to rest at the top of your head, and visualize the Mercury center as a nine-inch sphere of sparkling white light. Imagine this resplendent white light bursting with life-giving divine energy. Continue to focus on the white sphere of Mercury for some time.

10. Bring your attention back to the Saturn center at the base of the spine, and see the red glow. Quickly move your focus up through the other centers, visualizing each color in turn: red, violet, green, yellow, blue, indigo, and white. Endeavor to see all of the centers simultaneously as seven colored lights along the spine, neck, and head.

11. Release all visualizations, and meditate quietly for a few moments. When you are ready take three deep breaths and open your eyes.

WEEK TWO MEDITATION

The Center of the Sun

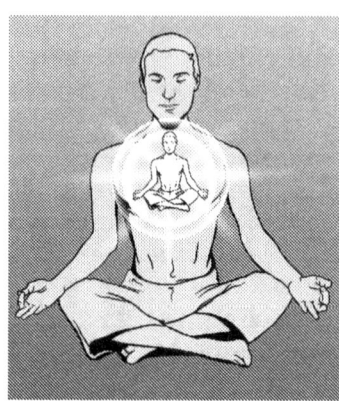

1. Perform the *Four Count Breath* and *Relaxation Exercise*.
2. Perform the *Purifying Light* meditation.
3. Close your eyes. Create an image of yourself about the size of your thumb, and see yourself in this small form sitting in the *Lotus Pose*. Shift your awareness into the Sun center in your heart, and visualize the small image of yourself seated within this center. Move your consciousness into your small form so that you see and experience yourself fully within the Sun center.
4. When this experience is steady, visualize a brilliant golden light descending in a downward spiral from far above the head of your larger physical body. From your position in the Sun center, look upward and watch this radiant golden spiral enter into the top of the head and continue downward into the spine of the physical body.
5. When the golden light reaches the heart, see it entering into the top of the head of your miniature body and filling your small form as you sit within the heart.
6. See your entire small being filled with and permeated by the descending golden light. Remain immersed in this luminous golden light, with your consciousness

firmly centered in the small being in the heart for several minutes.
7. To end the meditation, keep your awareness within your small form in your heart, and visualize the endless, subtle movement of a double spiral of white light moving up and down your spine, just behind you.
8. After a few moments, shift your consciousness into your head, just behind your eyes, and let go of the image of the small self. Stop all visualization, and meditate quietly for as long as you like, sensing golden energy radiating outward from the center of the heart, and integrating into every cell and molecule of your body. When you are ready, take three deep breaths, and open your eyes.

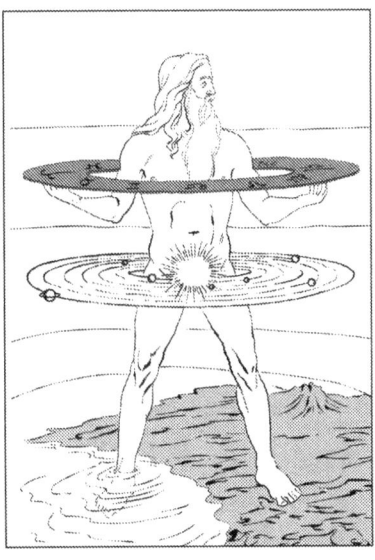

"The only beings on this earth... who are consciously alive and active within Spirit's inmost realm... are the Luminaries, the Bearers of Eternal Light."
Bô Yin Râ[48]

Living Light

WEEK THREE MEDITATION

Regenerating Light[49]

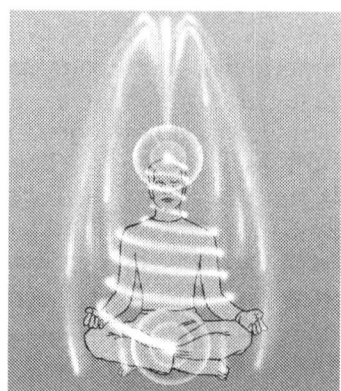

1. Perform the *Four Count Breath* and the *Relaxation Exercise*.
2. Perform the *Purifying Light* meditation.
3. Close your eyes and focus on the Saturn center at the base of your spine. Imagine a sphere of brilliant white light radiating out from this point.
4. Visualize and feel a wide beam of light coming out from the Saturn center. Imagine this ribbon of light moving upward around the outer edges of the body in a clockwise direction, wrapping the body tightly in bands of white light. The light should spiral upward, surrounding and encasing your body like a mummy.
5. When the band of light reaches the Mercury center at the top of the head, visualize the radiant light forming another brilliant, white sphere. As the light of this sphere intensifies, imagine a powerful projection of intense white light shooting upward, three feet above your head.
6. Imagine that this projection of light is like a fountain, and see sparkling light flowing downward into the aura surrounding your body. See and feel the fountain of glittering, vibrant, living light raining down all around you.

Living Light Meditations

7. When the light stream reaches the floor, let it cease. Once again see the ribbon of light emanate out of the sphere in the Saturn center. Watch the wide band of light wrap the body in an upward spiral, increasing the speed of its movement each time.
8. When the ribbon enters the sphere at the top of the head, again see it project upward into a fountain of radiant liquid light that streams down all around you. Repeat the movements of the upward spiral and the downward fountain for five to ten minutes.
9. End the visualization with a final flow out of the fountain overhead. Sit quietly for several minutes and feel the energy in your body. Be gently aware of sensations such as tingling or vibrations on the surface of the skin or within your body.

Note: It is helpful to memorize steps 3 through 9, and practice them a few times before proceeding with the next part of the meditation. The meditation may also be ended at this point if a shorter practice period is necessary. The remainder of the meditation can be added when you are ready. The complete meditation should be done as often as time allows during Week Three of Living Light.

10. When you are ready, visualize a wide beam of radiant white light coming out of the sphere in the Saturn center, and moving up the left side of the body. See the light pass through the sphere of the Mercury center, and then continue to flow down the right side of the body, passing through the sphere at the base of the spine, and continuing to flow up and down in a circle. Keep this light circulating from bottom to top, top to bottom, and side to side, creating a ring of moving light around the outside of the body.
11. When this image is moving steadily, visualize another beam of bright white light coming out of the Saturn sphere and traveling up the front of the body. See this stream of light pass through the sphere of Mercury, and flow down the back and through the lower sphere once again. Watch the light circulate from front to back as

you also see the other ring continuing to flow from side to side. The visual experience should be two rotating circles of light surrounding your body.
12. Imagine these two rings of light widening until they meet and form a solid sphere of moving light all around your body. See and feel yourself completely encased within the ascending and descending light for five to ten minutes.
13. To end the meditation, cease the circulation, and let the light return and dissolve into the Saturn center. Release all visual images, and quietly meditate while subtly noticing the physical sensations created by the movement of the light energy.
14. When you are ready, take three deep breaths, and open your eyes.

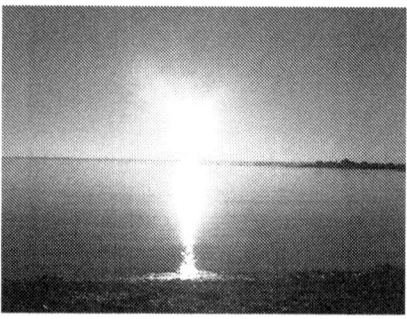

"The Light shines in the darkness..."
John, Ch. 1, Vs. 5

FASTING DAY MEDITATION

Fountain of Sustenance

This meditation is best performed outdoors in a private location in the sun within the first hour after sunrise. If weather conditions prevent one from going out or if the meditation is done later in the day, it should be practiced inside. It is only done once a week on fasting day. You should be seated cross-legged on the floor with the spine and neck in a straight line and the head centered over the tail bone.

1. Perform the *Four Count Breath* and *Relaxation Exercise*.
2. Perform the *Purifying Light* meditation.
3. Close your eyes and sit quietly for a few minutes, feeling the warmth of the sun on your head and body. If you are indoors, imagine that the sun is radiating down on you until you can feel its warmth.
4. Visualize the Mercury center at the top of your head as a sphere of intense white light.
5. Imagine a ray of sunlight coming down from the sun and entering into the sphere of white light at the top of your head. Imagine the Mercury sphere turning a brilliant white-gold as it receives this radiance from the sun.
6. See and feel the Mercury center becoming more and more alive with solar energy. Let the sphere expand and swirl with energy. See it spin and throw out glittering sparks of white-gold light.
7. Visualize a shaft of white-gold light descending from this sphere, entering into the top of your head and moving downward through your body. As it passes through the Moon center in the third eye, see this light expand into another sphere of dazzling golden-white light.
8. As the beam of light continues downward, and passes through the Venus center in the throat, see it again form a luminous white-gold sphere.
9. Follow the light as it enters into and fills the Sun center in the heart, creating another bursting sphere of golden

white brilliance. Let your awareness remain within the Sun center, and watch this sphere expand outward in every direction. Imagine a wide stream of sparkling light cascading downward from the heart. Watch the light immerse all of your internal organs, and fill the stomach, small intestines, colon, kidneys, liver, spleen, and reproductive organs with solar force. See the light flow out of the body through the anus and into the earth.
10. Imagine the solar light moving downward through the layers of the earth, and surging into its core. Inside the center of the earth, see a fiery ball of energy, a small and mighty sun. Let the golden-white light of the descending solar radiance merge with the inner earth sun.
11. Bring your awareness back up through the earth, visualizing the trail of light along the way. Let your attention rest within the Sun center in your heart. See and feel the light of the sun still flowing down into the top of your head, feeding you and filling you with light, love, and life. Remain in this awareness for several minutes.
12. When you are ready, visualize the light within the heart expanding outward again in every direction, permeating each cell and molecule of the body. Watch it emanate through all of the pores of the skin, filling the aura of the body and the surrounding area with flaming golden white sunlight.
13. Meditate on the vision of yourself immersed in this sphere of life-giving sunlight for several minutes. Turn your awareness to the feeling of the surface of the skin of your body where it contacts the air. Let your meditation quietly merge with this feeling.
14. When you are ready, imagine the ray of sunlight moving from the heart back up into the Mercury center at the crown of the head. Feel the warmth of the sun on the top of your head.
15. Cease all visualizations and meditate quietly for a while with open awareness and no thought.
16. When you are ready, take three deep breaths, and open your eyes.

Living Light Meditations

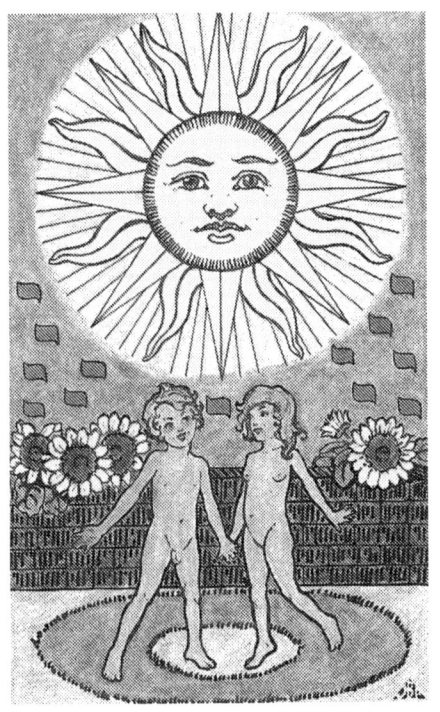

*"The wish, the heart's desire, the goal to be reached,
must be held firmly in mind, vitalized by divine power,
and propelled forward into the universe by the fiery
intensity of all the emotional exaltation we are capable of."*
Israel Regardie[50]

Chapter Six

Alchemical Yoga
Breath and Movement

THE RECONCILIATION OF BODY, MIND, AND SOUL

> *"This, thy body, O child of earth and sky, is truly the heavenly Vision of the Goodness of the Eternal. This, thy body is the Palace of the King; This, thy body is the manifested world of God and man; This, thy body is the seamless robe of ADONAI… and the Lord and His Temple are ONE."*
> The Book of Tokens[51]

A diet of raw and living foods, fasting on organic juices, and working with alchemical meditations fuel the inner fire that ignites the cellular impulse for transformative healing and growth. The meditations of *Alchemical Yoga* establish beneficial thought-forms that serve as patterns upon which a new and improved body may be built. Though the rewards to be gained by these practices are many, the energetic patterns they anchor in and around the physical form must be integrated into a receptive body. The body may be brought into a more open and subtle state by the regular practice of yoga.

Regular exercise, proper breathing, and the sacred consciousness induced by the focused movements of yoga are valuable keys that support the harmonious synthesis of all of the nutrition and energy that are derived from the Living Light diet and the powerful visual techniques of Alchemy. Yoga, which incorporates physical movements and stretches, breathing practices, mantra meditation, and a gently focused mind, offers special advantages over other types of exercise. The physical benefits that come from regular yoga practice are numerous and include increased flexibility, increased lubrication in the joints and connective tissues, improved muscle tone, decreased toxicity, and greater vitality. Yoga also impacts the mental and emotional natures, alleviating stress and soothing the soul.

As one works steadily in yoga practice, the body becomes purified, energized, and open. Hidden blockages are subtly released, transmuting deeply held resistances into states of peace and relaxation. During yoga, the attention is focused upon the breath, which is used consciously during movements and concentrated upon at rest. Another focal point is the mantra that is rhythmically repeated throughout each session. These techniques coordinate the body, mind, and soul as breath, mantra, and movement converge into deeply focused meditations.

The center point of the most powerful yoga traditions is the gentle, uninterrupted contemplation of the Brow Chakra. In Alchemy, this center of force is termed the Moon center and is associated to the pineal gland, which lies deep within the brain. In addition to the many powers that are attributed to this chakra, it is considered to be the command center for all of the cells of the body. When this center is properly charged, the rest of the body begins to spontaneously move toward greater balance and health.

In *Alchemical Yoga* the Moon center is energized through the symbol of a star. A star produces its own light deep within, and balances this inner fusion with outward radiance. Focusing on the imagery of starlight in the Moon center stimulates a similar process of light production within the pineal gland. This intense vibration is then emitted into the body, setting the course for cellular healing and regeneration. The star also reminds one that as one generates more light within the body, s/he may transmit healing vibrations for the benefit of others.

Alchemical Yoga integrates the visualizations and internal energy movements of alchemical meditation with the physical exercises and postures of Hatha and Kundalini Yoga. It also includes traditional breathing practices derived from various yoga philosophies and certain schools of Kabbalah. *Alchemical Yoga* taps into cosmic energies that emanate from both Western and Eastern streams of consciousness, instilling deep feelings of harmony and oneness while speeding rejuvenation.

Alchemical Yoga practices are easily learned and mastered; however, you should consult with a health care professional before beginning any new exercise program. During the Living Light program the introductory exercises, breathing techniques, and meditations described below should ideally be practiced daily, or at least two to three times a week. These practices support the body's natural cleansing process, and provide an opportunity to integrate the energy that is aroused through alchemical meditation into the cells of the body.

Choose an area for your yoga practice that is quiet, dust-free, and well-ventilated, and that allows sufficient space for you to stretch out fully on the floor. You will need a yoga mat, folded blanket, or pad. Wear comfortable, loose clothing, and no shoes or socks. Your stomach should be empty. Wait three hours after a full meal and ninety minutes after a light snack before beginning yoga. If you are practicing in the morning, be sure to drink some pure water on arising to help the body re-hydrate before yoga.

A warm shower before yoga practice will help the body open up and get the most from the yoga session. If you have long hair, roll it into a bun or knot and tie it on top of your head with a soft band. Do not burn incense nor play music during yoga practice. Let your session be a time of quiet inward focus that allows you to access and draw nourishment from the wellspring of all energy, all life that lies deep within.

Begin all of the practices seated on a mat in *Lotus*

Pose, Half-Lotus, or with your legs comfortably crossed in front of you. Straighten your spine and pull your neck in line, bringing the top of your head over your tailbone. Quiet your mind by focusing on your breath in its natural rhythm as it flows in and out of the body. On the inhale, mentally say the word, *I*. On the exhale, mentally say the word, *Am*. This *I-Am* chant may serve as a meditative breathing practice by itself, and it is also repeated mentally with each breath throughout the entire yoga session.

Work with all of the yoga poses and exercises according to your own needs in each moment. Do not force any movements. While you should feel a definite stretch, there should be no pain. If a posture is painful, bring yourself back to a point in the stretch or movement where the pain is relieved. Respect the limits of your body, and respond to its feelings. Listening to and following your own inner awareness is an important part of yoga practice. This guidance also applies to the breathing practices. Undertake breath work at your own pace, and stop when needed. You can always resume a breathing practice after a short break. Slow and steady progress is the goal in *Alchemical Yoga*.

BREATHING PRACTICES

Cleansing Breath

The *Cleansing Breath* greatly aids detoxification and helps clear the lungs and respiratory system. It is done three times before each *Alchemical Yoga* session, and may also be performed a few times each morning and evening.

1. Inhale deeply through the nostrils, feeling the breath descend and fill the body all the way to bottom of the spine.
2. Hold the breath in for a slow count of six.
3. Pucker your lips and forcefully exhale a little air through your mouth. This will create a whooshing sound.
4. Stop for a moment, and then force out a little more air.
5. Repeat the short sharp exhalations until all of the breath is exhaled completely.

Deep Breathing

Deep Breathing relaxes and energizes the entire body. It is done at the end of each yoga practice, and is very effective in helping to center one's energy at any time.

1. Inhale through the nostrils, bringing the breath into the upper chest and lungs.
2. As you continue to inhale, slowly move the breath downward, feeling the diaphragm expand.
3. At the fullest extent of the inhalation, the abdomen and lower back fill with the breath, and pressure is felt all the way down to the base of the spine.
4. Exhale through the nostrils slowly in reverse order, feeling the abdomen pull inward toward the spine.
5. Fully contract the diaphragm as the breath is completely exhaled.

Breath of Fire

Breath of Fire is one of the most renowned breathing practices in the yoga traditions of India. It cleanses and detoxifies the body and supports a healthy metabolism. In yoga, *Breath of Fire* is used during certain stretches and movements to improve one's flexibility and increase the effectiveness of the poses. This breathing technique purifies the blood and tones the nervous system. When *Breath of Fire* is combined with yogic exercises, it concentrates and increases the electromagnetic charge within the body, ultimately leading to inner stillness, blissful awareness, and *I AM* consciousness.

1. To perform *Breath of Fire*, exhale fully, and then begin to draw the breath in and out through the nostrils, maintaining a short quick exchange of air through the nose. When you place your hands on your diaphragm, you should feel it moving quickly in and out.
2. Continue to breathe in and out rapidly and rhythmically. You can adjust the breath, making it light or forceful, slower or more rapid. Do the *Breath of Fire* for one to three minutes to start, increasing to ten minutes over time. You may feel a bit light-headed when you first begin. Remember to work at your own pace.

Long Deep Breathing

Long deep breathing aids in lengthening one's extensions into yoga postures, and also restores emotional balance by releasing deeply held tensions and memories from the body. It has been referred to as *organic psychotherapy*[52] due to its ability to tap into and clear deep-seated blockages in the cellular structure of the body. You may feel anxiety or other emotions when engaged in long deep breathing. Recognize this as a cleansing of old emotional debris, and breathe through it smoothly.

1. Inhale slowly and deeply all the way to the base of the spine. Mentally chant *I*.
2. Exhale slowly all the way out. Mentally chant *Am*.
3. Continue long, deep, and slow, steady breathing while silently chanting *Iiiii-Aaaammm*.

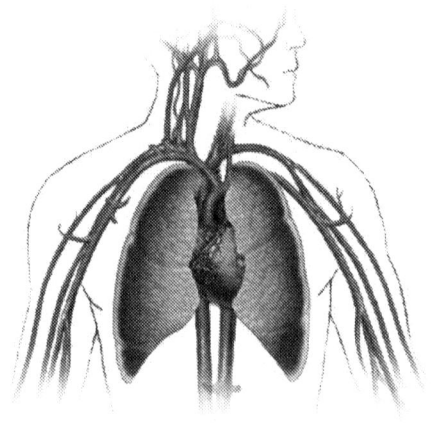

"An intelligent control of our breathing power will lengthen our days upon earth..."
Yogi Ramacharaka[53]

Bone Breathing

Bone breathing is an ancient Chinese healing practice introduced to the West by the Taoist master Mantak Chia in 1983.[54] It is a breathing meditation in and of itself, and is not used in conjunction with any yoga practices. It is offered for use during the Living Light program as a bonus practice that will increase your healing energy, and revitalize the body from the inside out. Try this practice at least one time during the Living Light program.

1. Sit comfortably and rest your arms on your lap. The palms of the hands are open and the fingers relaxed. Inhale gently through the nostrils into the lower abdomen. Exhale deeply all the way back out. Repeat this deep breath several times while relaxing. Return to normal breathing.
2. Focus your attention on the index finger of the left hand. As you naturally inhale, let your awareness along with the breath focus on a flow of energy moving from the tip to the base of the finger.
3. As you exhale normally through the nose let the energy stay in the finger and return your attention to the tip of the finger. Repeat the procedure with each breath.
4. As a sensation of heaviness or warmth develops in the left index finger compare it with the right index finger where you have not done any bone breathing yet. This will help you develop the ability to feel more deeply and identify the sensation that bone breathing brings.
5. As the left index finger becomes warmer or heavier expand the bone breathing into the rest of the fingers of the left hand, either one by one or all at the same time. As the left hand becomes warmer and heavier compare it with the right hand where no practice has been done yet.
6. Next incorporate the right hand into the practice by focusing on regular breathing and feeling the warmth and heaviness of the left hand moving into the right hand, or start working on the right hand finger by finger again.
7. Once both hands are feeling heavy continue the same practice, moving the energy of the breath up the arms

until the sensation reaches the shoulders.
8. For bone breathing through the feet it is best to remove the shoes and any tight clothing and guide your awareness up the toes, either singly or together up to the ankle.
9. For breathing up the spine begin at the tip of the sacrum and run your awareness up the spine higher and higher until you reach the base of the neck and the same feeling of warmth and heaviness is developed.
10. As the practice progresses and the body becomes relaxed, the noticeable breath through the nose may become more and more subtle. Do not try to force it back into greater awareness, rather let it stay subtle and calm. Continue to guide your attention into all of the bones.
11. Eventually it is possible to have the whole skeleton doing bone breathing, including the teeth. As practice develops try to breathe through the whole body at once, imagining that the bones are like a sponge absorbing the energy. You may refer to an anatomical chart of the skeleton to guide the energy with more precision.

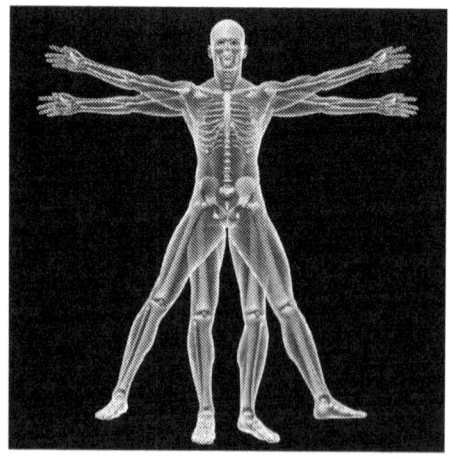

LIVING LIGHT ALCHEMICAL YOGA PRACTICE

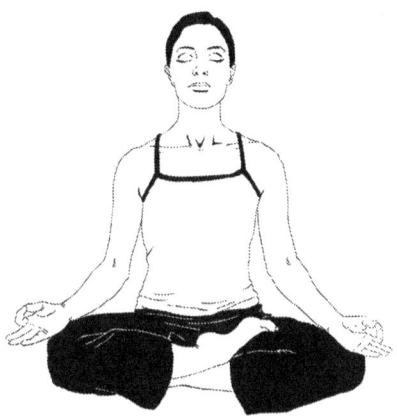

Half-Lotus Pose

* Sit in *Half-Lotus Pose*, cross-legged on the floor with your spine, neck, and head in line. Perform three Cleansing Breaths.

* Close your eyes and visualize a small, bright star within the Moon center at the level of the third eye, deep within the center of the head. While focusing on the star, mentally chant *I* silently with each inhale and *Am* on each exhale of the breath. Meditate in this way for several minutes until you can clearly see the star, and you feel centered and still in the *I-Am* breath.

* Stand up. Inhale while stretching the spine upward and raising your arms over your head. Extend the stretch as you inhale deeply.

* Exhale, bringing the arms down and folding forward at the waist. Let your hands drop toward the floor and hang for a few minutes. Fully release the neck and head, and allow the weight of your upper body to bring you deeper into the *Forward Bend*.

Living Light

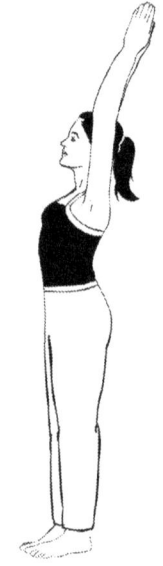 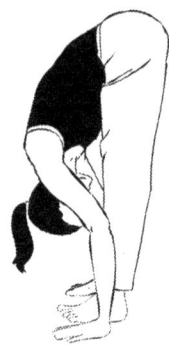

Overhead Stretch   **Forward Bend**

★ Inhale and come back up into the *Overhead Stretch* again.

★ Exhale back down into a *Forward Bend,* releasing the arms, head, and neck toward the floor.

★ Repeat the upward stretch and forward hang once more.

★ Perform three complete *Sun Salutes* following the illustration and instructions below:

Breath and Movement

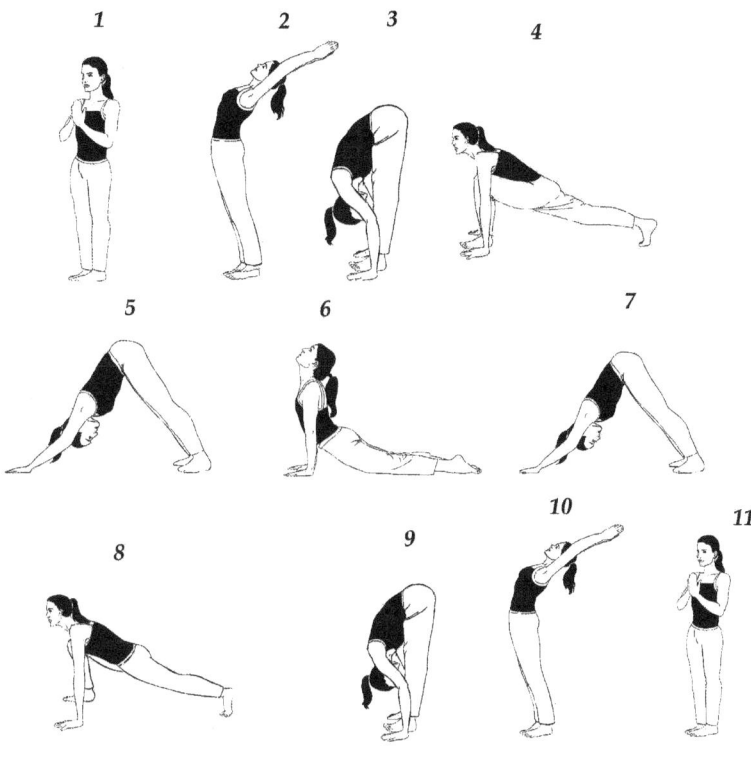

1. Stand up straight with your hands together in front of your chest in *Prayer Pose*.
2. Inhale while raising your arms overhead, keeping your hands together. Arch the back while extending the neck.
3. Exhale while bending forward until your hands reach as near to the floor as possible.
4. Inhale and bend your left knee and place your left foot flat on the floor between your hands. Exhale. Inhale and extend your right leg back, supporting your weight on the ball of your foot. Lift the torso upward, lengthening the spine. Lift the head and face forward. Hold this pose for a few minutes while focusing on the star and breathing *I-Am*.

5. On an exhale, move into *Downward Dog*. Place your feet and hands flat on the floor, and press your hips upward, keeping your head in line with your spine. Push the heels into the floor. Breathe deeply as you hold the pose for a few minutes.
6. On an inhale move to the floor and lie on your belly with your forehead on the floor and your hands beneath your shoulders. Exhale completely. Inhale and press up into *Cobra*, lifting your upper body up from the floor, and arching your back and neck. Keep your shoulders down.
7. Exhale and push back up into *Downward Dog*. Hold and breathe.
8. On an inhale bend your right knee and bring your right foot forward between your hands. Exhale. Inhale and extend your left leg back, supporting your weight on the ball of your foot. Lift the torso upward, lengthening the spine. Lift the head and face forward. Hold this pose for a few minutes while focusing on the star and breathing *I-Am*.
9. Inhale and stand up. Exhale and drop into a *Forward Bend*.
10. Inhale and stretch back up, raising the arms overhead, and coming into a backward arch.
11. Exhale and return to standing *Prayer Pose*.
12. Repeat the *Sun Salute* twice more.

* From standing *Prayer Pose*, inhale, and raise your arms up overhead. Exhale, lengthening the torso upward from the waist, and bending sideways to the left. Continue to reach up and over in *Blowing Palm*, and breathe deep and slow.

* Inhale, and return to the upright standing position. Exhale and release your arms letting them fall alongside the body.

* Inhale and bring your arms back up. Exhale and stretch your upper body to the right moving back into *Blowing Palm*. Hold and breathe for a few minutes.

* On an inhale, come back up. Exhale and release the arms.

Breath and Movement

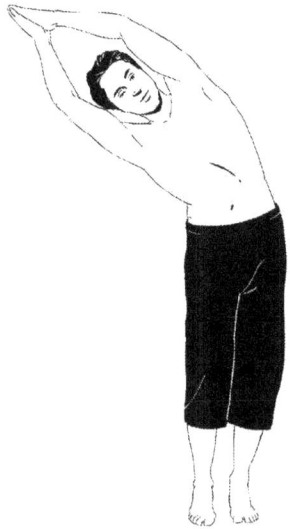

Blowing Palm

* Sit down on the mat in *Half-Lotus Pose*. Focus your awareness on the Mercury center at the top of your head. Visualize it as a sphere of brilliant white light. Inhale and bring a ray of this light down your spine into the Saturn center. Visualize the Saturn center at the base of the spine opening into a sphere of equally bright white light. Exhale and imagine a ray of light moving up the spine back into the Mercury center. Inhale and bring the light down the spine. Exhale and bring the light up the spine. Continue to breathe the light up and down between the spheres for a few minutes.

* Cease the visualization and meditate quietly, focusing your awareness on the star within the Moon center. Silently chant *I-Am* with each breath.

* Come into a cross-legged position, and hold your ankles with your hands. Close your eyes. Inhale and flex the spine, arching forward. Mentally chant *I*.

* Exhale and flex the spine backward, bringing it into an arch. Inwardly chant *Am*.

Living Light

* Continue to move the spine forward and backward, breathing and chanting *I-Am* for several minutes. Close your eyes as you move, meditate, and focus on the star.

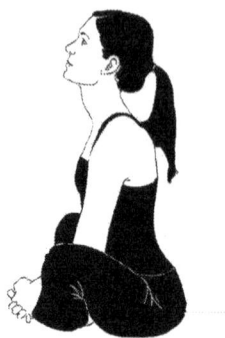 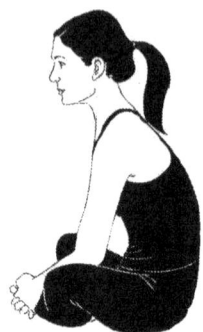

Spinal Flex

* Cease the movement. Return to *Half-Lotus Pose*, meditate on the star, and breathe *I-Am* for a few minutes.

* Let your arms drop down alongside your body. Close your eyes and continue to focus on the star as you inhale and stretch your neck upward. Exhale and let your chin fall toward your chest.

* Inhale and roll your head and neck counter-clockwise up over your left shoulder. Think about stretching up and out through the top of the head to keep the neck elongated throughout the roll.

* When your head reaches the top of your spine, exhale and continue to roll the neck downward across the right shoulder. When your chin comes to your chest, inhale and roll the head back up.

* Continue to move the neck in big *slow* circles while focusing on the star, breathing steadily, and silently chanting *I-Am*.

* After several minutes, cease the movement as the chin comes back to your chest.

* Reverse direction and continue slowly rolling the neck clockwise for a few minutes. Cease the movement as the chin comes to the chest. Inhale and raise your head.

* Return to *Half-Lotus Pose* and meditate quietly on the star for a few minutes while silently repeating *I-Am* with each breath.

* Come onto your hands and knees, keeping your face down and your head and neck in line with your spine.

* Remain in this pose and begin *Breath of Fire*. Close your eyes and focus your awareness on the star while you continue *Breath of Fire* for several minutes.

* Cease *Breath of Fire*. Remain on your hands and knees with your eyes closed, contemplating the star and breathing *I-Am* for a few moments.

* Inhale as you press your belly downward, and arch your head and neck backward.

* Exhale, arching your back upward, and bringing your chin into your chest.

* Continue the rhythmic breath and movement of *Cat-Cow* stretching for several minutes, mentally chanting *I-Am* with each breath.

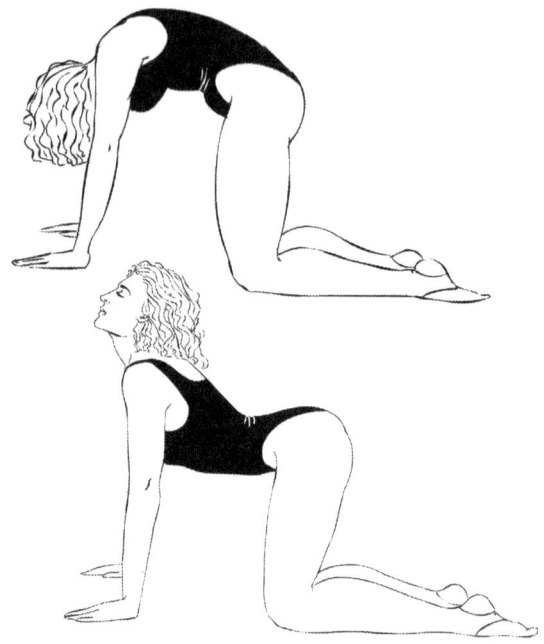

Cat-Cow Stretching

* Cease the movement, and bring your head and neck back in line with the spine and face downward. Remain on your hands and knees, close your eyes, and meditate on the star for a few minutes. Breathe *I-Am*.

* Sit back on your heels and place your forehead on the floor with your arms stretched out beyond your head and resting on the floor. Relax and close your eyes. Focus on the star and silently chant *I-Am* with each breath. Rest in *Child's Pose* for a few minutes.

Breath and Movement

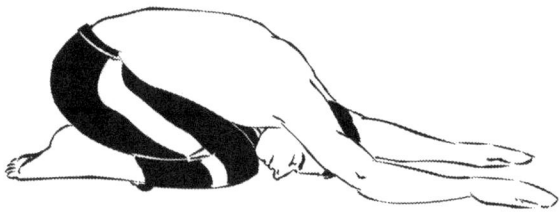

Child's Pose

* Slowly come up from *Child's Pose*, sit back on your heels again, and bring the spine up from the hips to the neck, one vertebra at a time. Rest your hands on your lap, and meditate for a few moments.

* Lie on your back, let your feet rotate outward, release your arms alongside your body, and completely relax. Meditate on the star while silently chanting *I-Am* with the breath.

* Bring your knees up to your chest. Grab your left knee with your right hand. Straighten the right leg onto the floor, and extend your left arm out from the shoulder. Bring your left knee across your chest, stretching the lower back and twisting the spine. Turn your head and neck, and stretch into the extended arm. Hold the stretch and breathe deeply.

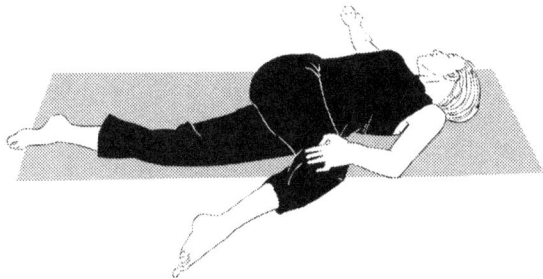

* Come back to center, stretch out, and relax for a moment. Bring your knees to the chest again, and

Living Light

repeat the stretch with the other leg. Return to center, stretch back out onto the floor and relax.

* Bend both knees, keeping your feet flat on the floor. Raise your left leg straight up from the hip. Flex the foot. Hold the toes of your left foot with your left hand, or place a strap across the foot, and hold the ends with your hand. Straighten your right leg and arm onto the floor.

* Begin *Long Deep Breathing*. Close your eyes and meditate on the star, breathing *I-Am* as you continue to press the leg and foot upward. Hold for several minutes, then release your leg onto the floor, and relax for a moment. Repeat the exercise with the right leg. Stretch back out onto the floor and relax. Meditate for a few minutes before continuing.

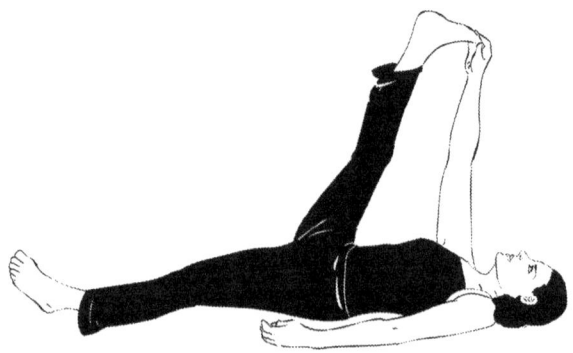

* Bring your knees into your chest and wrap your arms around your legs. Roll on your spine several times.

Breath and Movement

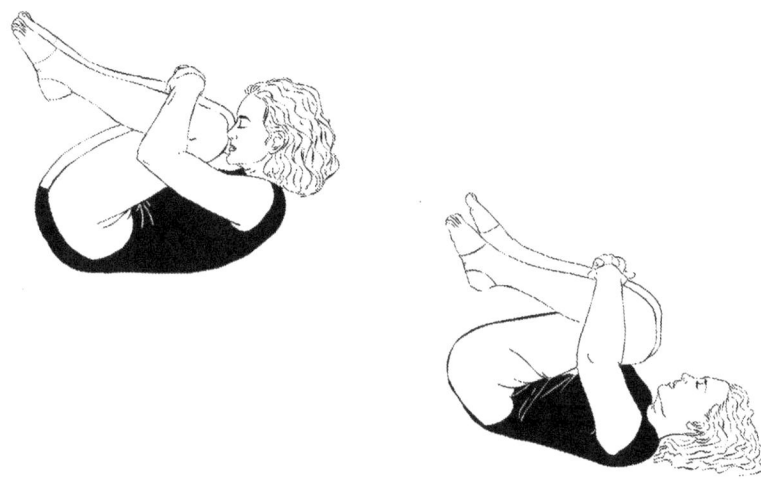

Spinal Roll

★ Return to *Half-Lotus Pose*, and meditate on the star while silently chanting *I-Am* with each breath for a few moments.

★ Place the soles of your feet together and hold your feet with your hands. Inhale deeply and stretch your spine upward. Exhale and bring your upper body forward and downward over your feet and arms. Stretch as far as you can into the pose. Perform *Breath of Fire* for several minutes while holding *Cobbler's Pose*.

Living Light

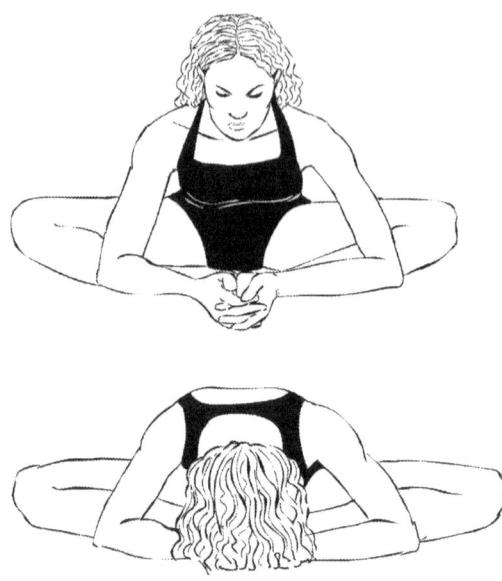

Cobbler's Pose

* Cease *Breath of Fire*. Inhale deeply and stretch as far as you can into the pose. Exhale and stretch as far as you can into the pose. Sit up into *Half-Lotus Pose*. Relax and meditate on the star, breathing *I-Am*.

* Take three deep breaths. Finish the session with meditation on *Lighting the Seven Lamps*.

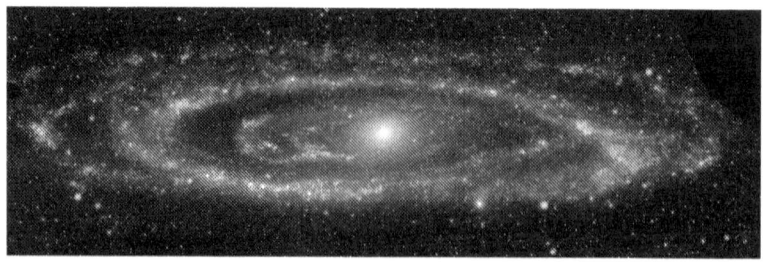

"Meditate on your Self, honor your Self, worship your Self, for God dwells within you as you."
Swami Muktananda[55]

Chapter Seven

Beyond Living Light

THE SECRET OF EQUILIBRIUM

Immersing oneself in a program of holistic regeneration for twenty-one days brings definite positive results. The body feels lighter, energy is restored, and peace of mind abounds. Now is a good time to carefully reflect on the new information that has been learned and plan for a future of abundant health and well being. It is not only possible but highly beneficial to continue to eat an 80 to 100% raw vegan diet.

The Living Light program initiates a process of deep cleansing within the body. The longer one follows the program, the healthier the body becomes. In certain illnesses and diseases it may make a critical difference in recovering health to continue to eat a 100% raw food diet that includes ample dark greens, super foods, and fresh, organic juices. This same approach is recommended for those who want to lose more weight. If one desires to return to eating some cooked foods, it pays to be selective about the type of foods that are cooked as well as the percentage of cooked foods in the diet.

Avoid falling back into the trap of processed and packaged foods. These things have little or no nutritional value. By the end of the Living Light program, the body is beginning to build a new and improved cellular structure using high quality, natural nutrition. When cooked foods are consumed, ensure they form no more than 20% to 30% of the diet, and consist primarily of steamed vegetables and whole grains.

Meat, dairy, and soy are best avoided or at least consumed only rarely, and in strictly organic forms. If at some point less desirable foods once again become a significant part of the diet, simply come back to Living Light, and cleanse and balance once more. Consciously take in the delicious freshness of raw foods in perfect harmony with healthy cooked foods. The list of foods to eat during preparation week given in Chapter Two offers an excellent dietary outline that will support a healthy and balanced life.

Maintaining the weekly 24-hour juice fast will support ongoing detoxification and regeneration by allowing the digestive system a chance to rest while the body cleanses away accumulated debris. This is also a good time to begin working with a three-day juice fast once a month. Within a few months one may choose to fast on juices for seven to ten days. If one feels ready, juice fasting may be extended for up to 90 days provided sufficient quantities of dark green vegetable juices are consumed.

Fasting is a divine technology of redemption that has a long history of healing virtually all imbalances and disorders. Fresh, organic vegetable juices contain superior nutrition in a highly absorbable form. Even when not fasting, juices should form an integral part of the regular diet in order to help maintain greater alkalinity in the body. Remember, the juice of green plants is liquid solar force that ignites the alchemical process of regeneration. As the cells are permeated with this transmuted sunlight, the body becomes super-charged with nourishment, energy, and bliss.

When one continues to eat a diet high in raw fruits, vegetables, nuts, and seeds, the body thrives. More energy is available for mental tasks and physical work. The Vital Essence of the plants of the earth keeps the cells in a purer state and youthfulness returns. The process of regeneration is aided over time by the proper balance of raw and cooked, whole and juiced, acid and alkaline, eating and fasting. This is the alchemical secret of equilibration as it applies to the physical body, the first aspect of the self that must be purified and transmuted in the transformative process known among alchemists as the *Great Art*.

When incorporated into one's life on a routine basis, exercise, yoga, and meditation are powerful allies in the quest for greater health, self-knowledge, and wisdom. Exercise accelerates breathing and heats the body, creating a true alchemical furnace that burns away toxic debris, fat, and gloom. Breathing practices also fan the sacred fire within, increasing the available Vital Essence. Through yoga the body becomes less rigid, more flexible, and slimmer while the mind becomes contemplative, peaceful, and sure. In the movement of the body and the pattern of the breath, find and embrace the balance point between active and passive, strong and flexible, rapid and still.

Meditation is a powerful tool for establishing and maintaining spiritual, mental, emotional, and physical equilibrium. The visual imagery used in alchemical meditation creates vibrant new thought-forms that establish more desirable patterns on the etheric plane. These forms are charged with spiritual light and anchored in and around the physical body, creating a new etheric foundation that stimulates ongoing refinements in the physical form.

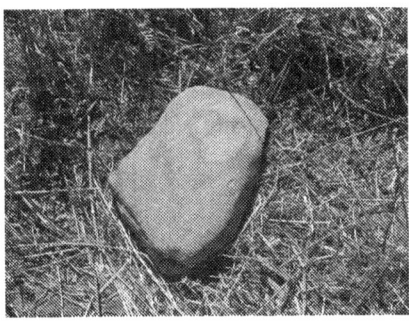

"You are the source of all that exists around you; you are the creator of your own world."
Osho[56]

In the Kabalistic view, the organic matter that constitutes the body only comes into being after the soul energizes a specialized matrix of light upon the etheric plane. The soul consciousness focuses imaginative energy and

Living Light

applies the higher will to attain a point of fusion in this light-body. When this critical mass of light energy is reached, dense matter is magnetized to the matrix and the physical body is born.

This principle underlies the alchemical teachings that creation is mental. Alchemical meditation techniques replicate the methods of the soul on the human level, and in doing so immediately brings one into an ever-expanding presence of the higher self. When the mind is focused on the flow of energy as it exists within the pattern of the soul, the physical body is drawn into greater alignment with the pure image of physical life intended by spirit. As practice continues, the connections between the etheric and physical bodies are strengthened, and improvements to the physical body come about more quickly. It is wise to make time to consciously work the balance between intellect and imagination, mind and emotions, body and soul.

THE ALCHEMY OF LIFE

Living and flourishing on a diet rich in natural raw food goodness doesn't mean becoming isolated from family, friends, and a social life. The raw vegan lifestyle is gaining prominence every day as hundreds of thousands of people discover the health benefits derived from raw foods. Raw food restaurants and cafes have sprouted around the world. This increased awareness has also spread to natural food supermarkets, health food stores, and even some grocery chains, which now stock items that support the raw vegan way of life.

Family members and friends who are not familiar with the raw food diet may be curious about how it works. Talk about your new diet with significant others but be wary of seeking too strongly to convert them in your enthusiasm. New ideas take time to root and grow. As your health, figure, and demeanor improve, others will see a living example of the rewards of a raw food diet that is far more powerful than words.

There is an abundance of excellent medical and scientific information about the positive health benefits of raw foods and juices that may also be of interest to friends and family members. Don't hesitate to share your knowledge and experience when asked, and point others toward raw food resources such as the Living Light plan. Just remain aware that the important act of helping others must be equilibrated with intentional devotion to one's own ideals and goals. Consciously balance the energies of service and attainment, love and will, self and others.

Integrating a high raw diet into an active lifestyle is easy. Have fun exploring new restaurants especially those offering vegetarian, vegan, and raw food fare. When dining out elsewhere keep in mind that most restaurants offer a variety of salads that can serve as a healthy main dish, though you may want to take along your own fresh salad dressing. There are also many delicious gourmet raw food recipes that offer feasts fit for those special occasions and holidays. Dehydrated foods are a great way to take living foods along when traveling, hiking, or camping. Below are a few bonus recipes to help you get started.

It is easy to maintain a healthy balanced lifestyle when you surround yourself with like-minded people. Many communities around the world offer raw vegan potluck dinners that provide an opportunity to meet others and share the delights of raw food dishes. See the Appendix for raw vegan festivals, gatherings, and Internet networks that can help you connect with raw food enthusiasts in your local community.

Regular spiritual fellowship helps keep the inner fires burning and provides important support for a more conscious life. Meditation and yoga classes are good places to meet others who are interested in self-improvement and living a more spiritually balanced life. Check with your local community center, telephone directory, and the Internet for resources in your area.

Many aspects of life beyond the diet will naturally change as a result of repeating and continuing the Living Light plan. Many more people are now awakening into the powerful potentials of raw veganism. Many of these folks report feeling a deep affinity and resonance with this way of life. Spontaneous conversions to a raw food diet do occur; however, such dietary changes also often come about naturally in the course of practicing Alchemy and other spiritual disciplines.

Living Light

Rudolf Steiner described vegetarianism as the *evolution of humanity*, a diet that would someday dominate the world. He also taught that coming to eat a diet consisting only of fruits and vegetables is a natural result of the esoteric growth process.[57] Be aware of the true meaning of these ideas. Though improving one's health with a better diet is always a wise undertaking, spiritual liberation cannot be attained through diet alone. Yet when such a state is attained, the diet naturally shifts to subtle, living foods.

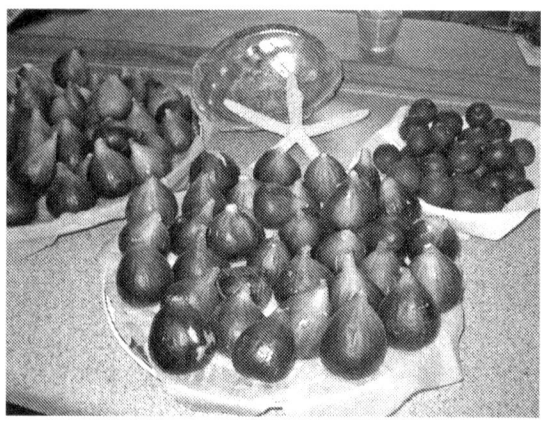

"Oh, to be the pure flawless crystal which lets Thy divine ray pass without obscuring... Not from a desire for perfection, but so that Thy work may be done as perfectly as possible."
The Mother[58]

BONUS RECIPES
HOLIDAYS AND SPECIAL EVENTS

Elegant Holiday Nut Loaves

1 C pecans, soaked
1 C walnuts, soaked
1 T fresh or ½ T dried rosemary
1 T fresh or ½ T dried thyme
1 T fresh or ½ T dried sage
1 clove garlic, minced
½ medium onion, chopped finely
2 stalks celery, chopped finely
1 red bell pepper, chopped finely
Flax oil as needed

Purée the nuts by processing them through a homogenizing juicer using the blank screen, or in a food processor using the 'S' blade. Place nut mix in a large bowl and add all ingredients, mixing with enough flax oil to form thick dough. Mold the mixture into small loaves and dehydrate at 105° F / 40° C for six hours. Serve warm with *Cranberry Sauce* (see Chapter Four for recipe). Alternatively, form the mixture into 1" rounds and serve fresh on lettuce.

Wheat Berry Summer Salad

2 C sprouted white wheat berries
1 C chopped celery
2 small fennel bulbs, chopped finely
1 C sunflower greens
½ C chopped parsley
¼ C chopped mint
6 large green olives, pitted and chopped
¼ C olive oil
4 T apple cider vinegar
Mineral or sea salt to taste
Ground black pepper to taste
Fresh field greens

Combine all ingredients except field greens in a large bowl and mix well. Refrigerate for one hour or more before serving on a bed of fresh field greens.

Heavenly Egyptian Fig Cakes

2 C dried figs
1 C walnuts, soaked
1 C almonds, soaked and roughly chopped
½ orange
Pinch of ground nutmeg
Pinch of ground cloves
Honey for dipping

Process the figs and walnuts in a homogenizing juicer using the blank screen, or in a food processor using the 'S' blade. Place fig and nut meal in a large bowl, and add the juice of ½ orange, 1 T of grated orange peel, nutmeg, and cloves. Mix well. Form mixture into 2" x 2" square cakes. Spread honey onto all sides of each cake, and dip in chopped almonds. Place cakes on a plate, cover, and refrigerate for one hour before serving.

Almond Nog

4 C thick *Almond Milk* (See Chapter Four for recipe)
1-inch length vanilla pod, soaked
1 T fresh ground nutmeg
Ice as needed

Place all ingredients in the blender and process, adding ice as needed to create a thick, frothy drink.

TRAVEL AND CAMPING

Canyon Trail Mix

½ C almonds, soaked
½ C sunflower seeds, soaked
½ C pumpkin seeds, soaked
½ C raisins, soaked
½ C cranberries, soaked
½ C Goji Berries, soaked
Mineral or Sea Salt to taste

Place soaked nuts, seeds, and fruits in a large bowl, add a little salt, and mix well. Place mixture on a dehydrator sheet and dehydrate at 105° F/ 40° C for two hours. Store trail mix in a sealed container.

Spirulina Energy Bars

1 C fresh dates
½ C raisins, soaked
½ C walnuts, soaked
½ C sunflower seeds, soaked
6 T Spirulina
Mineral or sea salt to taste
Golden flax seeds, ground

Process dates, raisins, and walnuts in a homogenizing juicer using the blank screen, or in a food processor using the 'S' blade. Place mixture in a large bowl and add remaining ingredients, using Flax seed meal as needed to make thick dough. Form mixture into 3" x 1" bars and place on dehydrator trays. Dehydrate at 105° F/ 40° C for six to eight hours. Store Energy Bars in an airtight container.

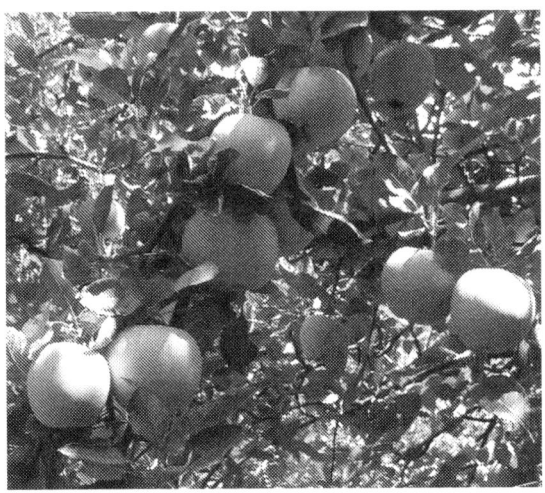

*"Come healing playing laughing with us miraculous ones.
Tickle us. Touch us. Heal us. Hold us dear.
We are always with you. We are always here."*
Susun S. Weed[59]

Veggie Rolls

4 carrots
4 stalks of celery
4 radishes
2 cucumbers
¼ C sunflower greens
1 avocado, mashed
Nori sheets
Mineral or sea salt to taste
Ground black pepper
  to taste

Finely slice carrots, celery, radishes, and cucumbers. Spread mashed avocado on Nori sheets. Top with sliced veggies, sunflower greens, and salt and pepper. Roll up the Nori, sealing the end with a little water.

Camp Soup

½ C carrots, shredded
½ C zucchini, shredded
¼ C celery, diced
½ C broccoli, diced
¼ C cauliflower, diced
½ C onion, diced
½ C red bell pepper, diced
5 sundried tomatoes,
  finely chopped
1 T dried mixed herbs
Mineral or sea salt to taste
Ground black pepper
  to taste
2 C water

Place all ingredients in a pot and add warm water (no more than 120° F/50° C). Stir well. Cover the pot and let stand for 30 minutes to 1 hour. The soup may be gently reheated to 105° F/ 40° C if needed before serving.

REACH YOUR LIMITLESS POTENTIAL WITH *ALCHEMICAL YOGA*®

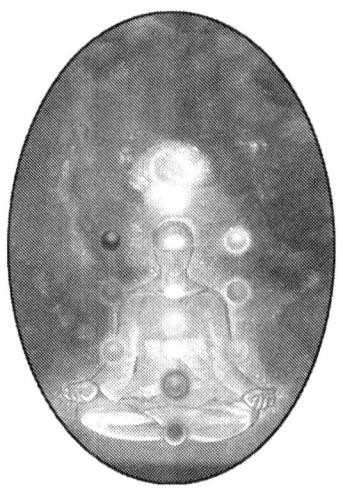

The Evolution of the Western Occult Traditions

"Man has a visible and invisible workshop. The visible one is his body, the invisible one his imagination…The imagination is a sun in the soul of man acting in its own sphere (the body), as the sun in our system acts on the earth. Wherever the sun shines, seeds planted in the soil grow, and vegetation springs up. The imagination acts in a similar manner in the soul, and calls forms of life into existence…The Spirit is the master, imagination the tool, the body the malleable material. Imagination is the power by which the will forms entities out of thoughts. It can produce and cure disease."

Thus Paracelsus, the renowned 15th century alchemist and philosopher, summed up the philosophy behind the magical arts of Alchemy. This basic premise, that the powers of human imagination bring all things to life in the body in the same way the sun calls forth life from the seeds of the plants on earth, has been an inherent part of the teachings of Western occultism for thousands of years. In Western occult schools, the alchemical secrets regarding the full potentials and proper use of the human faculties of imagination, will, mind, and spirit have been quietly preserved.

Modern occult teachers have continued to restore, clarify, and renew the ancient alchemical principles, interpreting much of the philosophy in psychological and physical terms. Significant among these leaders were Dr. Francis Israel Regardie and Paul Foster Case.[60] Dr. Regardie was the first modern occultist to externalize the teachings of the 19th century Order of the Golden Dawn, an organization whose founders and teachers were distinguished members of the European elite. Case also spent time with this order prior to establishing his own school of ageless wisdom, Builders of the Adytum (B.O.T.A.).

Though Regardie's act of publishing the previously secret materials of the Order of the Golden Dawn was scandalous at the time, today he is widely regarded as the most significant contributor to the present renaissance of occult magic. Dr. Regardie was a lifelong student of occultism, a professional chiropractor, and a distinguished practitioner and teacher of the psychiatric treatment methods of Carl Jung and Wilhelm Reich among others.[61]

Reich, as noted in Chapter One, was a psychiatrist who rediscovered Vital Essence within the body, and termed it *Orgone energy*. In approaches to psychiatric treatment based on Reich's work, spiritual energy is awakened in the body and directed toward the removal of *armoring*, the symptoms of which include muscle tension, numbness, obesity, and pain. Armoring was conceptualized as a process wherein old emotional energy had became suppressed and imbedded in the tissues of the body. Armoring thus kept the events that had caused the painful emotions from coming into conscious awareness for resolution and healing.

The concepts and methods of Carl Jung also influenced Dr. Regardie's understanding and approach to interpreting the many archetypal symbols found in the teachings and practices of Alchemy, Kabbalah, and Egyptian Rosicrucianism. In much of his work, Regardie merged the streams of Western occultism and modern psychology, creating a powerful synthesis between spirit and psyche, body and soul, and magic and psychotherapy. His many books continue to spread the light of mysticism and inspire new generations of students and teachers.

A contemporary of Dr. Regardie's, Paul Foster Case was a noted occult leader who brought forth important new insights into the ancient wisdom of the West. A brilliant occult scholar and gifted musician, Case devoted his life to establishing a body of work that declares the true purpose of Alchemy to be nothing less than a radical transformation of the human body, emotions, and mind. For Case, the goal of all occult practice was to liberate human consciousness from its identification with the limited personality, and bring it into union with the true self that is divine.

Case elucidated the secrets of Alchemy, Kabbalah, and Rosicrucianism in modern and accessible terms, bringing illumination and understanding from numerous fields of study into these heavily veiled traditions. Among the threads of wisdom Case wove into his comprehensive system for human spiritual development were the philosophies and disciplines of Yoga, Buddhism, and esoteric Christianity. His published works continue to awaken and accelerate all who sincerely seek for the light of wisdom that is hidden deep within. The bulk of Case's extraordinary teachings are available only to members of B.O.TA.

The Creation and Philosophy of *Alchemical Yoga*

As a long-time student, practitioner, and teacher of Western occultism and Eastern yoga, I value the many rewards to be gained from each of these spiritual paths. More than twenty years of careful study, analysis, and application of these venerable teachings on enlightenment, combined with my professional expertise in the field of human psychology and long-term use of Essene dietary principles laid the foundation for the creation of *Alchemical Yoga*.

My experience led me to conclude that the spiritual empowerment, divine understanding, and enlightened life promised by Alchemy, Kabbalah, and Rosicrucianism only come about when combined with the healing and regenerative powers of raw foods, juices, and fasting. Hints that diet and internal cleansing are key elements in the *Great Art* permeate the ancient alchemical texts. Alchemical symbols also hold much information about the biological aspects of enlightenment for those who have knowledge of their traditional meanings.

The disciplines of pranayama and Kundalini yoga were also alluded to by the old alchemists though they were veiled with obscure language that was designed to protect the authors from persecution, and keep the unprepared seeker from moving too quickly into the powerful experiences brought about by these methods. Due to the tireless efforts of modern occult scholars, many of their words have been decoded, and transcribed into modern language. In *Alchemical Yoga*, these unveiled techniques have been reconciled with their Eastern counterparts, and reunited with nutritional wisdom drawn from Western sources.

Alchemical Yoga is an artful discipline that began within the depths of my profound mergence with the creative source in meditation. To apply its methods to healing and regenerating the body requires no special knowledge of Kabbalah, Alchemy, or Yoga. It is a modern spiritual technology for advancing human consciousness and potentials that can be used in conjunction with any religion or philosophy, or with none. It combines divine science and esoteric arts to stimulate, support, and sustain positive and inspired growth in every aspect of one's life.

Since the inception of *Alchemical Yoga*, I have taught these methods to numerous people around the world. They have had great success in applying them toward the improvement of everything from their physical bodies and inner states of mind to the outer circumstances of their daily lives. The theories and practices of this system of yoga are defined by seven distinct alchemical stages: Purification, Disintegration, Disengagement, Communion, Regeneration, Crystallization, and Illumination.

The Living Light program that has been presented in this book consists of several of the core disciplines used in Purification, the first stage of *Alchemical Yoga*. These practices detoxify the physical body, engage and strengthen the powers of the imagination, soothe the mind, and ignite the sacred fire within. The work of Purification begun with Living Light does not end here, but continues to be applied throughout all of the higher stages of alchemical development.

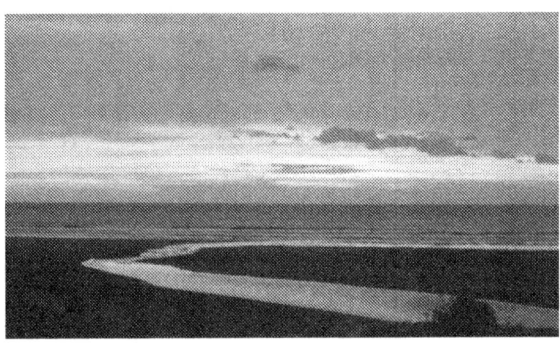

"Alchemical water...is the cosmic fire, specialized in the... chemistry of the blood stream. The purification of this water must be the first work of the alchemist. He must choose true foods and regulate his habits of eating... He must learn...to rebuild his body, sacrificing everything that clouds...its transparency to the Light..."
Paul Foster Case[62]

A wise master has said, "There is no perfection on this earth plane, only improvement." Therefore as long as the physical body remains on earth, the techniques of Purification must be applied to maintain the balance between life and death, darkness and light, spirit and matter. Only when the soul has been freed from earthly life, released its etheric form, and merged within the absolute unity of Kether, the crowning consciousness of *I AM,* do the impure side effects of manifestation finally disappear.

Alchemical Yoga is a holistic path encompassing self-improvement, a healthy lifestyle, and the possibility of extraordinary spiritual attainments. Its philosophy conceptualizes the human being as a dynamic convergence of spiritual force driven by one supreme consciousness that resides throughout the many higher dimensions of existence that lie beyond the physical world. The physical body is the only vehicle of this consciousness that is limited by the mechanics of the universe known as time and space.

In each of the remaining six stages of the yoga, the higher vehicles of the self are sought out, explored, and equilibrated using specific *Alchemical Yoga* techniques. The result of this work is the ongoing improvement of the mind, emotions, and soul that leads to greater spiritual awareness and the awakening of divine powers. In the subtle realms beyond the soul, contact may be made with the celestial essence of the true spirit, infusing the lower vehicles with the omnipotent consciousness of the creative source.

Even while such inspired goals are noted as future potentials, Alchemy returns again and again to the importance of the physical body as the living vessel that is necessary to anchor all of the higher bodies, and express the will of the spirit in life. Thus the alchemist continually seeks finer adjustments to the physical, mental, and emotional bodies that constitute the personality. In this way greater spiritual light may radiate into the world through the body and mind of the alchemist, making him or her into a living link between the supernal and terrestrial worlds.[63] Our greatest calling as alchemical yogini's and yogi's is to be a blessing to all we meet by manifesting the healing presence and love of the spiritual source in physical form.

When pursued with devotion, the higher levels of alchemical practice may one day enable one to receive nutrition directly from the sun, air, and earth as saints and yogi's are sometimes known to do. Rosicrucian alchemical teachings also direct attention toward the attainment of physical immortality. Greatly extended or eternal life is considered to be a valuable, spiritual advantage that allows the soul more time on earth to accumulate wisdom and attain divine life. Immortality grants respite from the otherwise endless wheel of death and rebirth which requires one to endure a great deal of conditioning in childhood that must be thrown off again and again in every incarnation in order to regain and access the knowledge of the soul.[64]

We live in a time of a great change and transformation wherein many people are awakening to the beauty, grace, and power that comes from living a spiritually informed life. *Alchemical Yoga* offers the opportunity to build upon the gains received through Living Light by applying the principles of purification, equilibration, and regeneration to each of the higher vehicles of the spirit in turn. This *Great Work* takes place steadily over time as new techniques are mastered and applied within each plane of consciousness.

Those who are interested in learning more about the higher applications of practical alchemy are invited to visit the web site of *Alchemical Yoga* at www.alchemicalyoga.com. To organize an *Alchemical Yoga* group in your local area, or for further information on available training, please write to training@alchemicalyoga.com.

Appendix

Living Light program CD

***Living Light: Alchemical Meditations for the 21-Day Regeneration Plan* by Chavah Aima**: On this companion CD to the book, Chavah Aima guides you through all of the key practices and visualizations used in the Living Light program. Relax and get the most from your alchemical practice with this convenient CD. The CD is $15.95 U.S., plus shipping, and may be purchased online at www.alchemicalyoga.com.

Recommended Reading

Raw Food Diet, Cleansing, Enzymes, Juicing, and Recipes

Survival in the 21st Century, *Sprout for the Love of Everybody*, and *The Lover's Diet* by Viktoras Kulvinskas, 21st Century Publications.

The Hippocrates Diet and Health Program and *The Wheatgrass Book* by Ann Wigmore, Avery Publishing.

Food Enzymes for Health and Longevity by Dr. Edward Howell, Lotus Press.

Cleanse and Purify Thyself, Books One and Two by Richard Anderson, N.D., Christobe Publishing.

Spiritual Nutrition, Rainbow Green Live-Food Cuisine, and *Conscious Eating* by Gabriel Cousens, M.D., North Atlantic Books.

Sprouts: The Miracle Food by Steve Meyerowitz, Sproutman Publications.

Heinerman's Encyclopedia of Healing Juices by John Heinerman, Prentice Hall Press.

Fresh Vegetable and Fruit Juices by Norman W. Walker, D.Sc., Norwalk Press.

Kundalini Awakening, Alchemy, and Meditation

Kundalini and *The Play of Consciousness* by Swami Muktananda, Siddha Yoga Publications.

Kundalini and the Evolution of Consciousness by Solomae Sananda, Living Spirit Press.

The Tower of Alchemy by David Goddard, Weiser Books.

Tao and the Tree of Life by Eric Yudelove, Llewellyn Publications.

Concentration by Mouni Sadhu, Wilshire Book Company.

Meditation as Medicine by Dharma Singh Khalsa, M.D., Atria Press.

RAW VEGAN COMMUNITY AND INTERNET RESOURCES

Living and Raw Foods: The largest community on the Internet dedicated to educating the world about the power of living and raw foods. www.rawfoods.com.

All Raw Times Home Page: The first web site for raw fooders since 1995. www.rawtimes.com. Check out their listings for restaurants, groups, and events.

Raw Vegan Radio: A radio show that will open your mind to holistic health, nutrition, and the connection between body, mind, and spirit.
www.rawveganradio.podomatic.com.

Meet Up®: Whatever your interest. Wherever you are. Enter "raw food" and "raw vegan" under Interest to find potluck dinners, and other events in your area. www.meet-up.com.

Raw Spirit Festival: The Grandest Raw Vegan, Eco-Peace Celebration on Earth. An annual event held in Sedona, Arizona, U.S.A. featuring a variety of inspirational presentations by international experts in raw food nutrition, gourmet raw food meals prepared by expert chefs, and much more. www.rawspirit.com.

RECOMMENDED SUPER-FOOD BLENDS

Green Vibrance® by Vibrant Health, www.vibranthealth.org.

Vitamineral Green® by Health Force, www.healthforce.com.

Greens Plus® by Orange Peel Enterprises, www.greensplus.com.

WHEAT GRASS GROWING KITS AND JUICERS

The Organic Wheat Grass Kit by Wheatgrasskits.com, www.wheatgrasskits.com.

Soil-less Wheat Grass Grower by Fern's Nutrition, www.fernsnutrition.com.

Miracle® MJ-550 Electric Wheat Grass Juicer and *Miracle® MJ-445 Manual Wheat Grass Juicer* available at several Internet retail outlets.

Samson® Multi-Purpose Juice Extractor, Samson Juicers, www.samsonjuicers.com, or call 1-888-992-7333.

RESOURCES FOR KITCHEN EQUIPMENT

Samson® Multi-Purpose Juice Extractor, by Samson Juicers, www.samsonjuicers.com or call 1-888-992-7333.

Bron® Professional Model H.D. Mandoline, top of the line mandoline and chef-quality slicers available at www.chefdepot.net.

Matfer® Mandoline, a reasonably priced simple-to-use mandoline, available at several Internet retail outlets.

Saladacco® Spiral Slicer, available at several Internet retail outlets.

Cuisinart® Food Processors, available at www.chefdepot.com and department stores.

Kitchen-Aid® Food Processors, available at several Internet retail outlets and department stores.

Vita-Mix® Blenders, available online at www.vitamix.com.

Excalibur® Dehydrator, available online at www.excaliburdehydrator.com.

COLON CLEANSING SUPPORT

Cleanse 28 by Arise and Shine, www.ariseandshine.com.

The Colon Cleansing Kit by Blessed Herbs, www.blessedherbs.com.

Dr. Christopher Cleansing Kit (Program #1), available through Health Force, www.healthforce.com.

Appendix

International Association for Colon Hydrotherapy
P.O.Box 461285
San Antonio, Texas 78246, U.S.A.
Phone: (001) 210-366-2888
Fax: (001) 210-366-2999
www.i-act.org

ENDNOTES

[1] *Leaves of Morya's Garden, Book II, Illumination,* Agni Yoga Society, 1925.

[2] *Alchemical Yoga*® is the registered trademark of the vital new philosophy and lifestyle discipline for personal transformation created by Reverend Chavah Aima. Please visit www.alchemicalyoga.com for more information.

[3] "The cause why I have painted these…in the form of Dragons, is because their stench is exceeding great, and like the stench of them, and the exhalations which arise within the glass, are dark, black, blue, and yellowish…the force of which…is so venomous, that truly there is not in the world a ranker poison; for it is able by the force and stench thereof, to mortify and kill everything living." Nicholas Flammel in *His Exposition of the Hieroglyphicall Figures which he caused to be painted upon an Arch in St. Innocents Church-yard, in Paris.* London, 1624, available at http://www.levity.com/alchemy/flam_h3.html.

[4] *Aphorismi Urbigerani, Or Certain Rules, Clearly demonstrating the Three Infallible Ways of Preparing the Grand Elixir or Circulatum majus of the Philosophers,* London, 1690, available at http://www.alchemywebsite.com/urbigeri.html.

[5] *Diet for a New America* by John Robbins, H.J. Kramer Publisher, Reprint edition, 1998.

[6] http://www.nofishing.net/FishFeelPain.asp.

[7] *Conscious Eating* by Gabriel Cousens, M.D., North Atlantic Books, Berkeley, California, 2000.

[8] *The Gospel of Luke* Chapter 15, Verses 11-32, The New Testament.

[9] *The Essene Gospel of Peace, Book One,* Edmond Bordeaux Szekely, International Biogenic Society, 1981.

[10] Chapter 64, Egyptian Book of the Dead, quoted in *Egyptian Magic* by Florence Farr, Kessinger Publishing Reprint, Montana, U.S.A.

[11] *Vitamin D casts cancer prevention in new light* by Martin Mittelstaedt, Globe and Mail, April 28, 2007, www.globeandmail.com.

[12] See www.solarhealing.com for more information on HRM and his work with solar gazing.

[13] *The Rebirth of Witchcraft* by Doreen Valiente, Phoenix Publishing, 1989.

[14] *The Path of Practice: The Ayurvedic Book of Healing with Food, Breath, and Sound* by Bri Maya Tiwari, Motilal Banarsidass Publisher, Dehli, 2000.

[15] *The Play of Consciousness* by Swami Muktananda, SYDA Foundation, New York, 2000.

[16] *Living Foods* by Ronald Bradley, Townsend Letter for Doctors and Patients, October 2001, available at http://findarticles.com/p/articles/mi_m0ISW/is_2001_Oct/ai_78900840.

[17] *The Truth About Coconut Oil* by Joseph Mercola, http://www.mercola.com/2003/sep/13/coconut_oil.htm.

[18] Dr. Alexis Carrel, 1912 Nobel Prize Winner in Physiology and Medicine, quoted in: *The Lover's Diet* by Viktoras Kulvinskas, MS, 21st Century Publications, 1997.

[19] *Daughters of the Goddess: The Women Saints of India* by Linda Johnsen, Yes International Publishers, Minnesota, 1994.

[20] http://www.qni.com/~gic/herb/barley.htm.

[21] *The Prophet* by Kahlil Gibran, Pan Macmillan, London, 1991.

[22] http://www.shirleys-wellness-cafe.com/bee.htm.

[23] *The Mistletoe and Its Philosophy* by P. Davidson in: *The Secret Teachings of All Ages* by Manley P. Hall, Philosophical Research Society, 1988, Los Angeles, California.

[24] *Survival in the 21st Century* by Viktoras Kulvinskas, P.O.Box 2853, Hot Springs, AK 79571, www.youthing101.com.

[25] *The Essene Gospel of Peace* by Edmond Bordeaux Szekely, International Biogenic Society, 1981.

[26] Extract from the *Gnostic Papyrus*, discovered in Egypt by James Bruce and preserved in the Bodleian Library in Oxford, quoted in *Egyptian Magic* by Florence Farr, Reprint by Kessinger Publishing Co., Montana, U.S.A.

[27] *The Sophia of Jesus Christ* in *The Nag Hammadi Gospels, The Nag Hammadi Library in English*, James M. Robinson, General Editor, Harper Collins, 1990.

[28] *The Protein Myth* by Physician's Committee for Responsible Medicine, Washington, D.C., www.pcrm.org.

[29] www.soyonlineservice.co.nz.

[30] *The Tree of Life* by Israel Regardie, Samuel Weiser, Inc., 1998.

[31] *The Miracle of Fasting* by Paul Bragg, N.D., PhD and Patricia Bragg, N.D., PhD, Health Science, Santa Barbara, CA.

[32] *Your Head in the Tiger's Mouth: Talks in Bombay with Ramesh Balsekar*, Zen Publications, Mumbai, India, 1998.

[33] *The Book of Thoth* by the Master Therion (Aleister Crowley), Ordo Templi Orientis, 1994.

[34] *Cleanse and Purify Thyself, Book One* by Richard Anderson, N.D., N.M.D., Christobe Publishing, Medford, OR, 2000.

[35] *Ozar 'Eden Ganuz* by Rabbi Abraham Abulafia, in *The Mystical Experience in Abraham Abulafia* by Moshe Idel, SUNY Press, 1988.

[36] *La Methode de'oraison Hesychaste*, A Biography of Symeon the New Theologian, in *The Mystical Experience in Abraham Abulafia* by Moshe Idel, SUNY Press, 1988.

[37] *The Book of the Sons of Fire, Chapter Three, The Brotherhood,* in *The Kolbrin,* Hope Trust, New Zealand, 1994.

[38] *Spiritual Nutrition and the Rainbow Diet* by Gabriel Cousens, M.D., Cassandra Press, California 1986.

[39] *The Kybalion: Hermetic Philosophy* by Three Initiates, The Yogi Publication Society, 1940.

[40] *Aesch-Mezareph, The Book of Purifying Fire,* translated by a Lover of Philalethes, 1714, in *Collectanea Hermetica* edited by W. Wynn Westcott, reprinted by Kessinger Publishing, Montana, U.S.A.

[41] This discussion of Alchemy reflects my interpretations and applications of the *Great Art* for the purposes of healing and physical regeneration. As presented in this book, it represents a basic introduction to alchemical science and practice. See Chapter Seven for more information on the philosophy and practices of Alchemical Yoga, including a brief review of some of the advanced work of Alchemy. Also visit www.alchemicalyoga.com.

[42] The etheric plane is theorized in Western occultism to be a field of energy surrounding and permeating everything in existence. This invisible substance is equivalent in function to the Kabbalistic world of Yetzirah, wherein patterns are made in astral light that form the foundation for physical form. This phase of creation is followed by the appearance of matter that constitutes the final world of Assiah, the plane of material life. The etheric body is the same energetic essence serving the same foundation-building function for the physical body.

[43] *An Introduction to Alchemy* by S.S.D.D. (Florence Farr), in *Collectanea Hermetica* edited by W. Wynn Westcott, reprinted by Kessinger Publishing, Montana, U.S.A.

[44] *The Kybalion: Hermetic Philosophy* by Three Initiates, Yogi Publication Society, 1940.

[45] *The True and Invisible Rosicrucian Order* by Paul Foster Case, Samuel Weiser, Inc., 1987.

Living Light

[46] *The Gospel of Philip* in *The Nag Hammadi Library*, James M. Robinson, Editor, Harper Collins, 1990.

[47] The perineum is located between the anus and the vaginal opening in women, and between the anus and the base of the penis in men.

[48] *The Wisdom of St. John* by Bô Yin Râ, translated from the German by B.A. Reichenbach, The Kober Press, Berkeley, California, 1975.

[49] *Regenerating Light* is an adaptation of the Body of Light technique introduced by the original Order of the Golden Dawn, and expanded upon by Israel Regardie in *The Art of True Healing* cited in (50) below.

[50] *The Art of True Healing* by Israel Regardie, edited by Marc Allen, New World Library, 1997.

[51] *Epilogos, The Meditation on Malkuth,* The Book of Tokens by Paul Foster Case, New and Revised Edition, Builders of the Adytum, Ltd., Los Angeles, 1989.

[52] *Kundalini Yoga* DVD by Ravi Singh and Ana Brett, www.raviana.com.

[53] *Science of Breath* by Yogi Ramacharaka, Yogi Publication Society, 1905.

[54] To learn more about Chinese Alchemy visit the website of Tao Master Mantak Chia at www.universal-tao.com.

[55] *Kundalini: The Secret of Life* by Swami Muktananda, SYDA Foundation, 1979.

[56] *The Book of Secrets* by Osho, St Martin Griffen, New York, 1974.

[57] *The Effects of Esoteric Development*, Ten Lectures at the Hague by Rudolf Steiner in 1913, Anthroposophic Books, 1997.

[58] *Sri Arurobindo and The Mother: Glimpses of Their Experiments, Experiences, and Realizations* by Kireet Joshi, The Mother's Institute of Research and Motilal Banarsidass Publishers, Delhi 1996.

[59] *Wise Woman Herbal: Healing Wise* by Susun S. Weed, Ash Tree Publishing, Woodstock, NY, 1989.

[60] Dr. Francis Israel Regardie, November 17, 1907-March 10, 1985. Paul Foster Case, October 3, 1884-March 2, 1954.

[61] *Israel Regardie*, biographical article by Chic and Tabitha Cicero, 1997, available at http://www.hermeticgoldendawn.org/Documents/Bios/regardie.htm.

[62] *Esoteric Keys of Alchemy* by Paul Foster Case, Ishtar Publishing, Vancouver, 2006.

[63] *An Introduction to Alchemy* by S.S.D.D. (Florence Farr), in Collectanea Hermetica, edited by William Wynn Westcott, Reprinted by Kessinger Publishing, Montana.

[64] *Raja Yoga* by Swami Vivekananda, Ramakrishna-Vivekananda Center, Revised edition, 1980.

BIBLIOGRAPHY

Agni Yoga Society. *Leaves of Morya's Garden, Book II, Illumination*, 1925.

Anderson, Richard, N.D., N.M.D. *Cleanse and Purify Thyself, Book One*, Christobe Publishing, Medford, OR, 2000.

Balsekar, Ramesh. *Your Head in the Tiger's Mouth: Talks in Bombay with Ramesh Balsekar*, Zen Publications, Mumbai, India, 1998.

Bô Yin Râ. *The Wisdom of St. John*, translated from the German by B.A. Reichenbach, The Kober Press, Berkeley, California, 1975.

Bragg, Paul, N.D., PhD and Bragg, Patricia, N.D., PhD. *The Miracle of Fasting*, Health Science, Santa Barbara, CA.

Case, Paul Foster. *The Book of Tokens*, Builders of the Adytum, Los Angeles, New and Revised Edition, 1989.
    Esoteric Keys of Alchemy, Ishtar Publishing, Vancouver, 2006.
    The True and Invisible Rosicrucian Order, Samuel Weiser, Inc., 1987.

Cousens, Gabriel, M.D. *Conscious Eating* North Atlantic Books, Berkeley, California, 2000.
    Spiritual Nutrition and the Rainbow Diet, Cassandra Press, California, 1986.

Farr, Florence. *Egyptian Magic*, Kessinger Publishing Reprint, Montana, U.S.A.

Gibran, Kahlil. *The Prophet*, Pan Macmillan, London, 1991.

Hall, Manley P. *The Secret Teachings of All Ages*, Philosophical Research Society, 1988, Los Angeles, California.

Hope Trust. *The Kolbrin*, New Zealand, 1994.

Idel, Moshe. *The Mystical Experience in Abraham Abulafia*, SUNY Press, 1988.

Joshi, Kireet. *Sri Arurobindo and The Mother: Glimpses of Their Experiments, Experiences, and Realizations*, The Mother's Institute of Research and Motilal Banarsidass Publishers, Delhi, 1996.

Johnsen, Linda. *Daughters of the Goddess: The Women Saints of India*, Yes International Publishers, Minnesota, 1994.

Kulvinskas, Viktoras. *Survival in the 21st Century*, P.O.Box 2853, Hot Springs, AK 79571.

Muktananda, Swami. *Kundalini: The Secret of Life*, SYDA Foundation, 1979.
    The Play of Consciousness, SYDA Foundation, New York, 2000.

Osho. *The Book of Secrets*, St. Martin Griffen, New York, 1974.

Ramacharaka, Yogi. *Science of Breath*, Yogi Publication Society, 1905.

Regardie, Israel. *The Art of True Healing*, edited by Marc Allen, New World Library, 1997.
    The Tree of Life, Samuel Weiser, Inc., 1998.

Robbins, John. *Diet for a New America*, H.J. Kramer Publisher, Reprint edition, 1998.

Robinson, James M. *The Nag Hammadi Library in English*, Harper Collins, 1990.

Steiner, Rudolf. *The Effects of Esoteric Development*, Ten Lectures at the Hague in 1913, Anthroposophic Books, 1997.

Szekely, Edmond Bordeaux. *The Essene Gospel of Peace, Book One*, International Biogenic Society, 1981.

Three Initiates. *The Kybalion: Hermetic Philosophy*, The Yogi Publication Society, 1940.

Therion, The Master (Aleister Crowley). *The Book of Thoth*, Ordo Templi Orientis, 1994.

Tiwari, Bri Maya. *The Path of Practice: The Ayurvedic Book of Healing with Food, Breath, and Sound*, Motilal Banarsidass Publisher, Dehli, 2000.

Valiente, Doreen. *The Rebirth of Witchcraft,* Phoenix Publishing, 1989.

Vivekananda, Swami. *Raja Yoga*, Ramakrishna-Vivekananda Center, Revised edition, 1980.

Westcott, W. Wynn. *Collectanea Hermetica,* reprinted by Kessinger Publishing, Montana, U.S.A.

Weed, Susun S. *Wise Woman Herbal: Healing Wise,* Ash Tree Publishing, Woodstock, NY, 1989.

INDEX

Adept, 119, 195
Alchemy, 1-4, 7-9, 11-12, 15, 17, 24, 28, 117-120, 122-123, 125, 144, 166-167, 173, 174-176, 178-179
Alchemical Angels, 13
Alchemical Demons, 12
Alchemical Meditation, 2-4, 24, 55, 59, 63, 64, 74, 118, 121, 123, 129, 143, 145, 165-166
Alchemical Yoga, 3-5, 11, 25-26, 28, 56, 117-118, 120-121, 125, 129, 143-146, 151, 173, 175-179
   Creation of, 175
   Stages of, 176
   Living Light Practice, 151
Alchemist, 2-3, 9-11, 13-15, 18, 118-119, 164, 173, 176-178
Alkalizing Broth, 83
Almond Cream, 85
Almond Milk, 85
Almond Nog, 170
Almond Seed Pâté, 94
Antipasto Treats, 92
Apple Nutmeg Delight, 112
Apple Pear Juice, 80
Avonaise, 75
Banana Coconut Fruigurt, 102
Banana Coconut Smoothie, 83
Banana Sundae, 114
Barley Grass, 32, 39, 41-42, 46
Basil Bean Salad, 87
Bean and Corn Salsa, 77
Bee Pollen, 32, 39, 43-44
Beet Relish, 107
Berry Fruigurt, 103
Black Dragon, 12
Blowing Palm, 154-155
Bone Breathing, 149-150

Bonus Recipes, 169
Breads, 104
Breakfast Dishes, 100
Breath of Fire, 147
Breathing Practices, 9, 27, 144-145, 146-147, 165,
Broccoli and Apple Salad, 89
Brow Chakra, 144
California Coleslaw, 87
Camp Soup, 172
Candida Overgrowth, 36-37
Canyon Trail Mix, 170
Cat-Cow Stretching, 157-158
Center of the Sun Meditation, 134-135
Chakras, 8, 10-11, 118-119
Cherry Vanilla Trail Mix Bars, 112
Child's Pose, 158-159
Chips, 104
Chlorella, 32, 39, 40, 42
Chocolate Chip Cookies, 113
Chocolate Covered Strawberries, 113
Chocolate Fudge, 111
Cilantro Carrot Soup, 91
Cleansing Breath, 146, 151
Cleansing Reactions, 16, 39, 52, 57, 63
Cobbler's Pose, 161-162
Colon Cleansing Kits, 53
Colonic Hydrotherapy, 19, 52-54
Concentration, 24-26, 122-125, 127-128
Corn Chips, 104
Crackers, 104
Cranberry Sauce, 76
Creamy Cilantro Dressing, 78
Creamy Sweet Potatoes, 92

Creamy Tomato Soup, 91
Crispy Pickles, 108
Cucumber Avocado Soup, 91
Cucumber Dill Salad, 90
Date and Walnut Cake, 115
Deep Breathing, 25, 56, 147
Desserts, 111
Detoxification Symptoms, 18-19
Diced Apples and Raisins, 101
Dips, 75
Dressings, 75
Dried Fruit and Seed Granola, 101
Drinks, 80
Elegant Holiday Nut Loaves, 169
Enema, 19, 53-54
Enzymes, 18, 32, 35, 38, 40, 42, 44, 48, 49, 58, 63, 65, 74
Equilibration, 119, 163, 164, 179
Essene Bread, 105
Etheric Body, 2-3, 118
Everyday Detox Juice, 82
Exercise, 4, 9, 19, 27-28, 56, 62, 65, 73, 74, 120, 129, 144-147, 165,
Extraordinary Mushroom Pâté, 97
Falafel Balls, 95
Fasting, 3, 8, 15-19, 32, 64, 143, 164, 176
Fasting Day, 64, 72, 83, 129, 139
Fasting Day Meditation, 139
Fermented Foods, 37, 107
Flax Crackers, 104
Fountain of Sustenance Meditation, 139
Four Count Breath, 128
Fresh Fruits with Super Seed Mix, 100
Friends and Family, 166
Garden Salad, 89
Garlic Seed Bread, 106
Great Art, 3, 12, 164, 176
Great Work, 119, 179
Greek Salad, 88
Green Dragon, 12-13
Green Lion, 17
Growing Greens and Grasses, 46-47, 52
Guacamole Dip, 78
Half-Lotus Pose, 146, 151
Healing Juice, 80
Heavenly Egyptian Fig Cakes, 170
Herbal Laxatives, 19, 53, 62, 63
Hermetic Philosophy, 122-123
Holidays and Special Events, 111, 167, 169
Illumination, 2, 13, 118, 176
Imagination, 2, 24, 25, 26, 118, 119, 122-123, 125, 127, 166, 173-174, 176
Immortality, 3, 178
Interior Stars, 118-119
Italian Dressing, 79
Joy, 8, 29-31, 35, 120, 121
Juicers, 18, 41, 47, 48, 52
Juices, 1, 3, 8, 11, 13, 16-19, 32, 35, 36, 38, 39, 47, 48, 52, 55, 62, 63, 64, 74, 80, 143, 163, 164, 166, 176,
Jupiter Center, 119, 132
Kabbalah, 1, 3, 4, 7, 8, 9, 11, 24, 26, 27, 145, 174-176
Kitchen Equipment, 47
Kundalini, 2, 9-10, 119,
Lighting the Seven Lamps Meditation, 132
Live Caesar Dressing, 80
Live Lasagna, 98

Living Light Program CD, 129, 181
Long Deep Breathing, 148, 160
Lunch Tacos, 95
Main Dishes, 94
Mantra, 23, 144
Mars Center, 119, 132
Mega-Green Juice, 81
Mercury Center, 119, 133, 136-137, 139-140, 155
Milks, 80
Mineral Magic Juice, 81
Miso Soup, 91
Mixed Berry Pie, 114
Moon Balls, 111
Moon Center, 119, 133, 139, 144, 151, 155
Morning Granola, 100
Non-Dairy Kefir, 86
Nori Crackers, 105
Nut Milk Preparation, 84
Ocean Salad, 89
Oils, 37-38
Orange Banana Fruigurt, 102
Organic Foods, 48-49
Orgone Energy, 8, 174
Our Daily Shred, 92
pH Balance, 63
Pizza Rounds, 99
Powerhouse Smoothie, 82
Pranayama, 27, 28, 176
Preparation Week Diet, 60
Preparation Week, 57-59, 83, 129, 164,
Preparation Week Meditation, 130-131
Preparation Week Sample Menu, 61
Probiotics, 36-37, 39, 42
Pumpkin Parmesan, 110
Purification, 36, 40, 41, 62, 117, 176-177, 179

Purifying Light Meditation, 129, 130-131
Raw Food Diet, 3-4, 15, 33, 63, 74, 163, 166-167
Raw Hummus, 76
Raw Raspberry Jam, 76
Raw Vegan Resources, 166-167, 182-183
Regenerating Light Meditation, 136-138
Regeneration, 1, 3, 4, 13, 15, 17, 26, 27, 29, 38, 40, 52, 57, 62, 74, 120, 121, 145, 163, 164, 176, 179
Reich, Wilhelm, 8, 174
Rejuvelac, 108
Relaxation Exercise, 128-129
Salads, 87
Sample Daily Schedules, 73
Sample Menu Plans, 66-72
Saturn Center, 119, 132, 133, 136-138, 155
Sauces, 75
Sauerkraut, 107
Sea Vegetables, 32, 35, 39, 42
Seed Cheese, 109
Serpent Power, 9, 119, 125
Sesame Kale Salad, 90
Seven Metals of the Alchemists, 118-119
Seven Planets of the Ancients, 118-119
Shopping List, 50-51
Side Dishes, 87
Smoothies, 80
Soak Times, 45-46
Solar Force, 14, 17, 140, 164,
Solar Gazing, 9, 11, 21-23
Soups, 87
Spaghetti Squash, 96
Spicy Mexican Salsa, 77
Spinach Caesar Salad, 88
Spinal Flex, 155-156

Living Light

Spinal Roll, 160-161
Spirulina, 32, 39-40, 42
Spirulina Energy Bars, 171
Spreads, 75
Sprouting Directions, 44-45
Sprout Salad, 88
Sprouts, 17, 32, 35, 44, 45, 52, 65
Summer Passion Juice, 81
Sun Salute, 152-154
Sunshine, 8, 20-23
Sunflower Seed Milk, 85
Sunlight Burgers, 96
Super-Food Powders, 42, 65
Super-Foods, 32, 39-44, 52, 62, 63, 74, 163
Super Green Smoothie, 83
Super Seed Mix, 109
Super Seven Juice, 81
Sushi Rolls, 98
Tabouli, 96
Tamari Dressing, 78
Tangy Tomato Dressing, 79
Thought-Forms, 122, 127, 143, 165
Tomato Basil Dressing, 79
Tomato Basil Salad, 90
Toppings, 109
Tossed Chinese Vegetables, 97
Transmutation, 2, 24, 117, 118
Travel and Camping, 167, 170
Treats, 111
Tropical Breakfast, 101
Turkish Flat Bread, 106
Veganism, 16, 167,
Vegetable Loaf, 95
Vegetarianism, 16, 168
Veggie Rolls, 172
Venus Center, 119, 133, 139
Vessel of Alchemy, 3, 11, 178
Visualization, 20, 26, 55, 122, 125-127, 128, 129, 145, 155, 181
Vital Essence, 2, 8-11, 13, 17, 23, 32, 38, 40, 48, 55, 62, 64, 117, 119, 123, 164, 165, 174
Vitamin D, 21
Walnut and Sun-Dried Tomato Pâté, 94
Wheat Berry Porridge, 102
Wheat Berry Summer Salad, 169
Wheat Grass, 16, 39, 40-41, 65
Yoga Practice, 3, 4, 9, 11, 19, 27, 28, 55, 56, 62, 63, 65, 73, 74, 118-119, 120, 129, 143-146, 151, 165
Zesty Marinara Sauce, 77

ABOUT THE AUTHOR

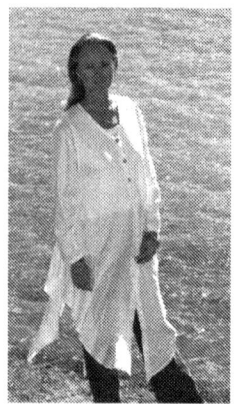

Reverend Chavah Aima is an Adept in the Western Mystery traditions, and a Yogini in the Eastern Yogic traditions. From childhood she has had a clear awareness of the multi-dimensional nature of existence, and has received spiritual visions and guidance from the celestial realms. Throughout her life, Chavah has been immersed in the mystical studies and practices of many different systems of spiritual expansion.

Chavah's desire to awaken and empower the divine being that lies within the human form inspires all of her work. She views all of life from the unified consciousness, transcending the appearance of duality that causes so much discord and disharmony in the manifest world. The mergence of her energetic connections to both the Western and the Eastern enlightenment traditions has resulted in the creation of the vital new discipline known as Alchemical Yoga. Alchemical Yoga offers studies and practices that bring about deep healing, peaceful serenity, and personal spiritual empowerment.

As an initiate of the esoteric arts and sciences, Chavah teaches Hermetic Kabbalah, Alchemy, Rosicrucian philosophy, the Egyptian mysteries, and Kundalini and Tantra Yoga. For nearly twenty years, she has advocated and taught the use of raw foods, juices, and fasting for healing and spiritual acceleration.

Chavah is the author of numerous magazine and Internet articles, and a comprehensive correspondence course that unveils the master within, which is offered through Heart of the Rose mystery school. She is the Founder and Executive Director of Enlightened Life Sanctuary, an international non-profit organization that encourages the wise use of our collective spiritual and material resources to consciously create sustainable and enlightened life on earth. For more information on the work of Reverend Chavah Aima, please visit her web sites: www.alchemicalyoga.com and www.enlightenedlife.org.

www.ingramcontent.com/pod-product-compliance
Lightning Source LLC
Chambersburg PA
CBHW070401240426
43661CB00056B/2496